Fast Facts: Thyroid Disorders
First published January 2006

Text © 2006 Gilbert H Daniels, Colin M Dayan
© 2006 in this edition Health Press Limited
Health Press Limited, Elizabeth House, Queen Street, Abingdon,
Oxford OX14 3LN, UK
Tel: +44 (0)1235 523233
Fax: +44 (0)1235 523238

Book orders can be placed by telephone or via the website.
For regional distributors or to order via the website, please go to:
www.fastfacts.com
For telephone orders, please call 01752 202301 (UK), +44 1752 202301 (Europe),
800 247 6553 (USA, toll free) or 419 281 1802 (Canada).

Fast Facts is a trademark of Health Press Limited.

A CIP record for this title is available from the British Library.

ISBN 1-903734-65-7

Daniels, GH (Gilbert)
Fast Facts: Thyroid Disorders/
Gilbert H Daniels, Colin M Dayan

Medical illustrations by Annamaria Dutto, Withernsea, UK.
Typesetting and page layout by Zed, Oxford, UK.
Printed by Fine Print (Services) Ltd, Oxford, UK.

Printed with vegetable inks on fully biodegradable and
recyclable paper manufactured from sustainable forests.

444   001
Low emissions
during production

Low   Sustainable
chlorine   forests

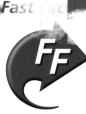

Fast Facts:
Thyroid Disorders

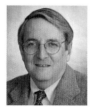

Gilbert H Daniels MD
Professor of Medicine
Harvard Medical School
Co-Director, Thyroid Clinic
Massachusetts General Hospital
Boston, Massachusetts, USA

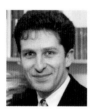

Colin M Dayan MA FRCP PhD
Head of Clinical Research
Henry Wellcome Laboratories for
Integrative Neuroscience and Endocrinology
University of Bristol, Bristol, UK

Declaration of Independence
This book is as balanced and as practical as we can make it.
Ideas for improvement are always welcome:
feedback@fastfacts.com

⊬ HEALTH PRESS

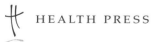

Glossary 4

Introduction 7

Thyroid physiology and function tests 9

Hyperthyroidism: etiology and presentation 26

Hyperthyroidism: diagnosis and management 41

Hypothyroidism: etiology and presentation 69

Hypothyroidism: diagnosis and management 79

Pregnancy and the thyroid 94

Thyroid nodules and thyroid cancer 109

Useful addresses 139

Index 140

Glossary

ACTH: Adrenocorticotropic hormone; a hormone secreted by the anterior pituitary gland that stimulates secretion of glucocorticoids by the adrenal cortex

Amiodarone-induced thyrotoxicosis: type 1 is induced by the high iodine content of amiodarone, and may be due to Graves' disease or toxic nodular goiter; type 2 is a form of destructive thyroiditis resulting from the toxic effects of amiodarone and/or its metabolites

ANCA: anti-neutrophil cytoplasmic antibodies

Athyreosis: congenital absence of the thyroid gland

Bruit: an intermittent, harsh or musical auscultatory sound

CEA: carcinoembryonic antigen (a tumor marker)

Deiodinase: several related enzymes responsible for conversion of T4 to active T3 (types 1 and 2) or to the inactive form of T3, reverse T3 (type 3)

Euthyroidism: normal function of the thyroid, in which the proper amount of hormone is secreted with correct constitution

Familial dysalbuminemic hyperthyroxinemia: a genetic disorder characterized by elevations in serum total thyroxine and (in some assays) free T4, caused by an abnormal serum albumin that has increased affinity for thyroxine

Follicular thyroid carcinoma: a well-differentiated thyroid carcinoma derived from follicular cells

G-CSF: granulocyte colony-stimulating factor

Goiter: an enlargement of the thyroid

Graves' disease: an autoimmune condition in which anti-TSH-receptor antibodies stimulate the thyroid and produce hyperthyroidism

Hashimoto's disease: a type of chronic autoimmune thyroiditis that may cause primary hypothyroidism

HCG: human chorionic gonadotropin, a hormone produced during pregnancy and in pregnancy-related states, which can mimic the action of thyroid-stimulating hormone on the thyroid

Hot nodule: an autonomously functioning thyroid adenoma that is defined by its enhanced ability to accumulate radio-iodine

Hydatidiform mole: an uncommon benign tumor that develops from placental tissue early in a pregnancy in which the embryo has failed to develop normally and secretes high levels of HCG

Hyperemesis gravidarum: excessive vomiting in early pregnancy

Hyperthyroidism: overproduction of thyroid hormone by an overactive thyroid

Hypothyroidism: underproduction of thyroid hormone by an underactive thyroid

Ishihara color charts: tests for color-blindness

Jod–Basedow effect: iodine-induced hyperthyroidism, which occurs particularly as a result of excess iodine ingestion/administration in patients with multinodular goiter

MALT: mucosa-associated lymphoid tissue, the origin of many marginal-zone, B-cell thyroid lymphomas

Multinodular goiter: a thyroid with more than one nodule

Myxedema: a generalized non-pitting swelling of the skin that occurs in profound hypothyroidism – not to be confused with pretibial myxedema; also a synonym for profound hypothyroidism

Papillary thyroid carcinoma: a well-differentiated, thyroid carcinoma derived from follicular cells

Pendred's syndrome: autosomal-recessive condition characterized by deafness associated with goiter and mild hypothyroidism

Pretibial myxedema: a rare non-pitting, disfiguring skin infiltration that generally involves the anterior tibial region and dorsum of the foot; seen in association with Graves' disease

Radio-iodine: radioactive isotopes of iodine (either ^{123}I or ^{131}I) taken up by thyroid tissue; can be used for thyroid imaging (^{123}I or ^{131}I), for imaging thyroid cancer (^{131}I) or for therapy (^{131}I)

Struma ovarii: ectopic thyroid tissue comprising the bulk of an ovarian teratoma; may cause hyperthyroidism

T3: triiodothyronine or liothyronine; active thyroid hormone produced mainly by deiodination of T4 in the peripheral tissues, with a small amount produced and released by the thyroid

T4: tetraiodothyronine or levothyroxine (or L-thyroxine); the major (precursor) hormone product of the thyroid

TBG: thyroid-binding globulin; the major thyroid-hormone-binding protein in the blood; also called thyroxine-binding globulin

THBR: thyroid-hormone-binding ratio; an inverse measure of the serum binding proteins for thyroid hormone from which the amount of free T4 can be estimated

Thionamides: a group of drugs including propylthiouracil, methimazole (prescribed in the USA) and carbimazole (prescribed in the UK), used to inhibit synthesis of thyroid hormones in hyperthyroidism

Thyroglobulin: a high molecular weight protein on which thyroid hormones are synthesized; the storage form of thyroid hormone (a key component of colloid in the center of the thyroid follicles); serum thyroglobulin is a tumor marker for well-differentiated thyroid carcinoma

Thyrotoxicosis: any condition attributable to excess circulating thyroid hormone levels

Toxic nodular goiter: a multinodular goiter producing excess amounts of thyroid hormone

TRH: thyrotropin-releasing hormone; produced by the hypothalamus; stimulates the pituitary to produce TSH

TSH: thyroid-stimulating hormone; produced by the pituitary; stimulates the secretion of T4 and T3 by the thyroid

Introduction

In recent years, thyroid function tests have become routinely available to almost all physicians. Clinical chemistry laboratories in the UK typically perform over 20 000 tests each year. This volume of testing is not unreasonable, given that abnormalities of thyroid function rival diabetes mellitus in terms of prevalence, and can affect any system of the body. In the UK and USA, palpable thyroid nodules are present in one in 20 of the population. As a result, all doctors can expect to encounter thyroid disease in one form or another.

Thyroid disorders can usually be managed satisfactorily, but there are traps for the unwary. The presentation of thyroid dysfunction is often atypical, particularly in the elderly. In addition, 'routine' thyroid function testing shows that subclinical thyroid disease is ten times more common than clinical disease – one in ten women in the UK and USA has subclinical disease – and this poses difficult questions of how and when to intervene. Similarly, ultrasonography shows that, worldwide, up to half of the population over 65 years of age has thyroid nodules.

Initiating treatment for thyrotoxicosis is relatively straightforward, but completing treatment to the patient's satisfaction can be more complex and can take several years. The management of thyroid disease during pregnancy and of thyroid eye disease poses particular challenges, while the effective treatment of hypothyroidism with thyroxine has recently been questioned by both researchers and patient groups.

In *Fast Facts: Thyroid Disorders* we aim to provide all the necessary information in a concise and practical format to enable the general physician to negotiate potential traps with confidence. Knowing when to test, when to treat and when to refer will result in the rapid initiation of appropriate therapy and, just as importantly, reduce the unnecessary anxiety that both physicians and patients feel when coping with these common conditions.

Thyroid physiology and function tests

Thyroid hormone synthesis and regulation

Synthesis and secretion. The thyroid is the main site of iodine uptake in the body, concentrating iodide from the blood against an electrochemical gradient through the action of the sodium iodide symporter, an internal membrane protein that resides in the thyroid epithelial cells. The enzyme thyroid peroxidase incorporates iodine into two hormones (Figure 1.1):

- liothyronine (containing three iodine atoms and also known as triiodothyronine or T3)
- levothyroxine (L-thyroxine; containing four iodine atoms and also known as tetraiodothyronine or T4).

T3 and T4 are stored in the form of thyroglobulin in the colloid of the thyroid follicles and are released when thyroid-stimulating hormone (TSH) from the pituitary gland stimulates the thyroid. T3 is the active form of the hormone; it has a shorter half-life (1 day) in the circulation than T4 (about 7 days). T3 binds to three thyroid hormone receptors, one that is largely restricted to the pituitary and two that are widely distributed.

The adult thyroid typically produces about 90 µg of T4 and 6 µg of T3 daily. More than 99% of circulating T4 and T3 is bound to protein: 70% of T4 is bound to thyroid-binding globulin (TBG; also known as thyroxine-binding globulin), 10–15% to thyroid/thyroxine-binding prealbumin (transthyretin) and 15–20% to albumin. When the concentration of binding proteins such as TBG increases or decreases, the serum concentration of T4 and T3 (which bind to these proteins) also increases or decreases, respectively. However, the free hormone concentrations remain normal.

Peripheral conversion of T4 to T3. About 80% of circulating T3 is produced enzymatically by the deiodination of T4 in peripheral tissues – mainly the liver and kidneys. T4 is converted to T3 in most tissues by two related enzymes, deiodinase types 1 and 2, while another enzyme, deiodinase type 3, converts T4 to an inactive form of T3 (called reverse T3 or rT3). Thus, replacement of thyroid hormone with T4 alone provides a long-lasting store of thyroid hormone that is gradually converted to T3, resulting in stable plasma levels of both T4 and T3.

Direct thyroid production of T3 may increase in patients with iodine deficiency and in those whose thyroid is overstimulated by TSH or by anti-TSH-receptor antibodies, as occurs in patients with Graves' disease. Starvation, severe illness and many drugs impair the peripheral conversion of T4 to T3, which may cause a decrease in the metabolic rate. It is uncertain whether the resulting decrease in overall metabolic rate is beneficial or harmful.

Feedback control. T4 and T3 production is controlled by TSH from the pituitary gland, which itself is controlled by thyrotropin-releasing hormone (TRH) secreted by the hypothalamus (see Figure 1.1). Increases in the levels of circulating thyroid hormone (T3 and T4) suppress both TRH and TSH, completing the negative feedback loop. The pituitary appears to be less sensitive to circulating T3 than to T4, suggesting that intrapituitary conversion of T4 to T3 may be a better way of delivering T3 to the pituitary than circulating T3 itself.

Serum TSH is exquisitely sensitive to small changes in serum thyroid hormone concentrations. For example, a 50% reduction in free T4 in the serum produces a ninetyfold increase in serum TSH concentration. The normal range of serum thyroid hormone concentrations is relatively broad; modest decreases or increases within this normal range indicate the earliest stage of thyroid disease and are reflected in serum TSH concentrations that move out of the normal range.

Iodine intake. The recommended daily intake of iodine for adults is 150–300 µg. Iodine levels can be measured in the urine, as this is the major route of iodine excretion. Iodine supplementation in the form of iodized salt is standard practice in many areas of the world, and many multivitamins also contain iodine, generally 150 µg/tablet.

Goiter, hypothyroidism and endemic cretinism are all significant risks when iodine intake falls below 50 µg/day. The highest iodine content is found in fish, with smaller amounts in milk, eggs and meat.

Iodine deficiency is typically due to the consumption of local produce in areas where the soil has a low iodine content such as high mountainous areas. Low iodine levels are also found in parts of Europe and lowlands situated far from the oceans. Mild iodine deficiency (intake < 100 µg/day) occurs in many Western European countries, but is uncommon in the UK, Switzerland or The Netherlands.

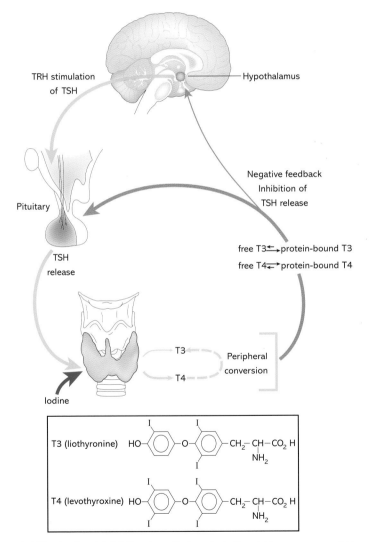

Figure 1.1 The feedback inhibition loop that controls thyroid hormone secretion.

In cases of mild iodine deficiency, thyroidal iodine uptake increases and the thyroidal secretion of T3 relative to T4 becomes greater than usual. Conversely, an excess of iodine triggers an autoregulatory process in which uptake of iodine by the thyroid decreases, secretion of thyroid hormone is inhibited and the ratio of secreted T4 to T3 increases.

Thyroid function tests

The main thyroid function tests are:
- TSH level (the most common first-line test)
- T4 (or free T4) level
- T3 (or free T3) level.

T4 (or free T4) assays are generally more robust and less prone to interference during intercurrent illness than measurements of T3. For this reason, the routine use of T3 assays is controversial. Nevertheless, as practice varies in different parts of the world, the interpretation of both T4 and T3 assays is discussed here.

In most cases, interpretation of thyroid function tests is straightforward (Figure 1.2). However, complex cases can occasionally be encountered, and the physician should be aware of the possible differential diagnoses (Table 1.1). Raised concentrations of protein-bound T4 and T3 in the blood occur when there are increased levels of binding proteins, for example in pregnancy and during estrogen therapy. However, serum TSH is normal in these circumstances; free T4 and free T3 are generally normal in these circumstances as well.

Discordant T4 and T3 results are unusual, but may be seen in severe non-thyroidal illnesses, in which the conversion of T4 to T3 is impaired. The antiarrythmic amiodarone is also a powerful inhibitor of T4-to-T3 conversion (see page 21). Patients taking T4 may present mildly discordant results (slightly high T4 and free T4, normal T3), while patients taking T3 may present markedly discordant results (high T3, low T4). High T4 and normal T3 may be seen in patients with familial dysalbuminemic hyperthyroxinemia, an inherited condition in which an abnormal albumin binds large amounts of T4 but not T3. Discordant results may also result from interference with one of the assays. Any such results should be discussed with the testing laboratory.

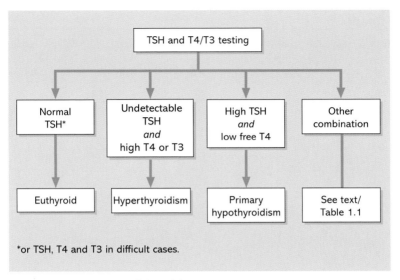

Figure 1.2 Interpretation of thyroid function tests.

First-line testing. A TSH assay that can detect less than 0.02 mU/L of TSH is widely recommended as the first-line thyroid function test, because TSH is a more sensitive indicator of thyroid dysfunction than T4 or free T4, and the assay is robust. In almost all cases, serum TSH concentrations can be interpreted as follows:
- low serum TSH indicates hyperthyroidism
- high serum TSH indicates primary hypothyroidism
- normal serum TSH indicates a euthyroid state.

However, an intact hypothalamo–pituitary axis is necessary for TSH to reflect thyroid status appropriately. When pituitary disease is present, serum TSH measurements must be interpreted in conjunction with free thyroid hormone concentrations. The normal (or sometimes slightly high) serum TSH level often seen in hypopituitarism is due to the production of a TSH molecule with intact immunologic but impaired biological activity. A missed diagnosis of hypopituitarism may prove fatal if, as a consequence, the associated hypoadrenalism is left untreated. Some endocrinologists believe that the risk of missing such cases is sufficiently high to justify routine measurement of T4 or free T4 in addition to TSH (although this view is controversial).

TABLE 1.1

Interpretation of thyroid function tests in patients with different clinical and biochemical measurements

	TSH	T4	True status
TSH normal, but patient not euthyroid			
Hypopituitarism (central hypothyroidism)	N	L	Hypothyroid
Transition from hyperthyroidism to hypothyroidism	N	L	Hypothyroid
Transition from hypothyroidism to hyperthyroidism	N	H	Hyperthyroid
TSH-secreting pituitary tumor	N*	H	Hyperthyroid
Thyroid hormone resistance	N	H	Variable; usually euthyroid
Abnormal proteins	N	H	Euthyroid[†]
Laboratory error	N	H or L	Hypothyroid or hyperthyroid
TSH low, but patient not clinically hyperthyroid			
Subclinical hyperthyroidism	L	N	Subclinically hyperthyroid
Severe non-thyroidal illness	L[‡]	N or L (free T3 is low)	Euthyroid**
Recently treated hyperthyroidism	L	N or L	Euthyroid or hypothyroid
High-dose glucocorticoid or dopamine therapy	L[‡]	N	Euthyroid
Central hypothyroidism (hypopituitarism)	L[††]	L	Hypothyroid
Use (abuse) of T3-containing therapy	L	L (isolated increases in T3)	May be hyperthyroid
Laboratory error	L	N	Euthyroid

*Or slightly raised; [†]In the absence of concomitant disease; [‡]Rarely completely suppressed; [††]Occasionally normal or slightly elevated.

Comment

TSH often surprisingly normal, particularly with hypothalamic disease. Note the possibility of associated hypoadrenalism requiring urgent treatment.

If TSH is suppressed for a long time, it can take weeks or months to respond to hypothyroidism (common after treatment of hyperthyroidism).

Rare transient situation, sometimes seen after excess thyroxine therapy for profound hypothyroidism, or after intermittent thyroxine use.

Rare.

Thyroid hormone does not stimulate its receptor. When resistance is present only at the pituitary level, the patient will be hyperthyroid.

e.g. excess TBG or dysalbuminemic hyperthyroxinemia.

Rare.

Common, especially in the elderly. May be due to high-dose thyroxine therapy. Associated with increased risk of atrial fibrillation and possibly osteoporosis. Management of endogenous subclinical hyperthyroidism is controversial.

Thyroid function tests should be repeated after recovery.

If T4 is low, the patient may actually be hypothyroid.

Transient. T4 or T3 may be low if the patient is also severely ill.

Hypothalamic disease may result in a pituitary that releases biologically inactive TSH, which is still detected in laboratory assay. Note the possibility of associated hypoadrenalism requiring urgent treatment.

T3 inhibits TSH, which prevents T4 production by the thyroid.

Rare.

**When severe, may represent central hypothyroidism;
H, high; L, low; N, normal.   (CONTINUED)

TABLE 1.1 (CONTINUED)

Interpretation of thyroid function tests in patients with different clinical and biochemical measurements

	TSH	T4	True status
TSH high, but patient not clinically hypothyroid			
Subclinical hypothyroidism	H	N	Subclinically hypothyroid (mild thyroid failure)
Recent treatment of severe hypothyroidism	H	N	Euthyroid
Recovery from severe non-thyroidal illness	H	N	Euthyroid
Adrenal insufficiency (primary)	H	N	Euthyroid
TSH-secreting pituitary tumor	H	H	Hyperthyroid
Heterophilic (interfering) serum antibodies	H	N	Euthyroid
Laboratory error	H	N	Euthyroid

H, high; L, low; N, normal.

TSH measurements alone may also be misleading if insufficient time has elapsed for thyroid function to equilibrate. Serum TSH reaches its nadir 5–6 weeks after an increase in T4 dosage, a fact that is particularly relevant for patients who take their thyroid hormone intermittently. Conversely, serum TSH may remain suppressed for weeks or months after treatment of hyperthyroidism. In these cases, free T4 and/or free T3 levels should be monitored until TSH is no longer suppressed.

Laboratory or clerical errors, or TSH assay interference arising from the presence of heterophilic antibodies, may also result in misleading TSH measurements.

Comment

Very common (occurs in 5–10% of women); usually autoimmune. May be associated with symptoms of hypothyroidism. Often treated with thyroxine.

It takes several weeks for TSH levels to reach a new level of equilibrium after treatment with T4.

Transient. Thyroid function test should be repeated after 1–2 months.

Low cortisol results in increased TSH release. Thyroxine therapy may precipitate adrenal crisis. Diagnose and treat hypoadrenalism urgently. Review thyroid function 1–2 months later, as it may be true thyroid failure.

Rare.

TSH is persistently high but T4 is not even slightly low. Discuss with laboratory. Result may change with a different assay. Not a laboratory error, but interference in TSH measurement from patient's serum.

Rare.

The scheme shown in Figure 1.3 is recommended when TSH alone is used as the first-line test. It can be adapted into a treatment algorithm by addition of suitable threshold values for TSH.

TSH reference ranges do not need to be adjusted for age in adults. However, values are up to four times higher in the first year of life, particularly in cord blood and in the first 3 days of life, and must be interpreted according to age-specific reference ranges during this period.

If TSH levels are abnormal, or any of the conditions shown in Table 1.2 is present, suspicion of thyroid disease should be high and additional thyroid function tests should be performed.

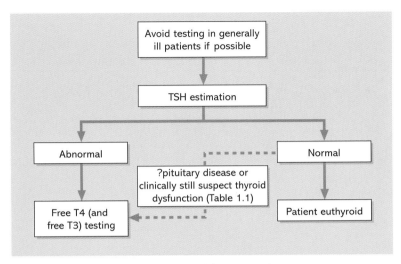

Figure 1.3 Suggested scheme for thyroid function testing.

Free and total hormone levels. Many laboratories now use assays for free, rather than total, T4 and T3, because they are less influenced by changes in the binding and transport of thyroid hormone. However, these tests are more expensive, and are more susceptible to interference by serum factors during severe illness. When total thyroid hormone assays are used, the free component can be estimated by adding radiolabeled T3 to serum and measuring the amount that binds to thyroid-hormone-binding proteins. This test is known as the T3 resin uptake (T3RU) or the thyroid-hormone-binding ratio (THBR), from which the free T4 index (FTI) can be calculated (the product of the T4 × T3RU or THBR). The THBR is reduced at high levels of binding protein and raised at low levels of binding protein. THBR measurement is used less often now that free T4 and T3 assays are more common.

Patient selection. A first-line thyroid function test should be carried out in:
- patients with a palpable goiter or nodule
- patients with classic symptoms of hyperthyroidism (weight loss, tremor, palpitations, heat intolerance, sweating)
- patients with classic symptoms of hypothyroidism (recent weight gain, mental slowing, cold intolerance, dry skin, constipation)

TABLE 1.2

Non-classic presentations of thyroid disease, indicating the need for thyroid function testing

Hyperthyroidism	Hypothyroidism
Weight loss alone	Carpal tunnel syndrome
Atrial fibrillation	Growth failure in children
Pyrexia of unknown origin	Galactorrhea (elevated prolactin)
Persistent vomiting	Recurrent miscarriage (anti-thyroid antibodies)
Hyperemesis gravidarum	
Unexplained cardiac disease, including congestive heart failure	Pregnant women with goiter or history of thyroid disease
Gynecomastia	Individuals with other autoimmune diseases
Osteoporosis	Individuals with premature hair graying (under 30 years old)
	All pregnant women at booking (controversial)

- patients with mild symptoms suggestive of thyroid disease and a family history of hyperthyroidism or hypothyroidism
- pregnant women, or those contemplating pregnancy, with any symptoms suggestive of hyper- or hypothyroidism, or with a family history of thyroid disease.

Although biochemical thyroid dysfunction is common, it may not be clinically apparent or may present in a non-classic way (see Table 1.2). Controversially, routine testing of all pregnant women was proposed by some, but not other, authorities after the publication of data suggesting that mild hypothyroidism may affect neurological function in offspring (see Chapter 6). The results of ongoing prospective studies in this area are awaited.

Patients with severe non-thyroidal illness. Metabolic changes during severe illness may make thyroid function tests very difficult to interpret.

Starvation or severe illness results in a fall in serum T3 concentrations, primarily because the conversion of T4 to T3 is inhibited. However, measurement of T3 is not a first-line test, so this rarely causes confusion in the clinical setting.

The acute phase of critical illness (usually when it is severe enough for the patient to require intensive care) may inhibit the release of TSH, and levels of serum T4 and/or free T4 fall below normal as a consequence. Under these circumstances, the subnormal serum TSH should not lead to the incorrect diagnosis of hyperthyroidism. Serum TSH generally remains detectable (even if subnormal) unless glucocorticoids or dopamine, which can both suppress serum TSH, are also used. In the recovery phase of the illness, the pituitary appears to recognize that the low free T4 concentration is abnormal, and serum TSH rises above normal (usually to less than 20 mU/L) until the free T4 level returns to normal.

Abnormal values of T3, T4 and TSH are seen in 50%, 15% and 10%, respectively, of hospital inpatients, and in a higher proportion of patients in intensive care. If possible, thyroid function testing should be postponed until after recovery, unless thyroid dysfunction is strongly suspected. Subtle changes should not be interpreted further, but certain marked changes are strongly suggestive of true thyroid dysfunction (Table 1.3).

Drug interference. Few drugs interfere with serum TSH measurements, but high-dose glucocorticoids or dopamine infusions may partially suppress serum TSH.

Alterations in binding and transport proteins. Estrogen (including that produced during pregnancy), tamoxifen, raloxifene, methadone and 5-fluorouracil increase binding-protein levels, while androgens and anabolic steroids reduce levels. Although free hormone measurements are generally normal in these conditions, marked alterations in binding proteins may slightly raise or lower free hormone levels. Salicylates, phenytoin and carbamazepam (carbamazepine) compete for T4 binding to transport proteins and reduce total T4, but seldom affect free hormone levels significantly. Heparin administration, and the use of heparinized tubes for blood collection, may cause false elevations of

TABLE 1.3

Informative results from thyroid function tests in patients with non-thyroidal illness

Assay finding	Interpretation
Normal or raised T3 or free T3 with undetectable TSH	Probable hyperthyroidism
Markedly raised TSH (e.g. > 20 mU/L)	Probable hypothyroidism
Normal TSH	Probable euthyroidism (if no pituitary disease)

free hormones by releasing free fatty acids, which displace the hormones from their binding sites. Serum TSH remains normal under these circumstances and can still reliably indicate thyroid status.

Amiodarone. The antiarrhythmic amiodarone is a powerful inhibitor of T4-to-T3 conversion, and usually elevates T4/free T4 levels while decreasing T3/free T3 levels. Mild TSH elevations may occur transiently. These changes rarely result in the misdiagnosis of thyroid disease if TSH levels are used as a first-line test. Amiodarone and several other drugs can precipitate true thyroid dysfunction (see Chapters 2, 3, 4, 5, 7), which should be distinguished from interference in thyroid function tests.

Additional biochemical thyroid tests

TRH stimulation test. This has been replaced by sensitive TSH assays in all but the most complex cases. TRH is not available in the USA.

Thyroid autoantibodies. Three autoantibody tests, which confirm the presence of autoimmune thyroid disease, are commonly available.

Anti-thyroid peroxidase antibodies, formerly called antimicrosomal antibodies, are present in 45–80% of patients with Graves' disease and up to 95% of patients with autoimmune hypothyroidism. Although not pathogenetic themselves, anti-thyroid peroxidase antibodies are the most readily available test of autoimmune thyroid disease and are useful for predicting prognosis in mild thyroid dysfunction.

Anti-thyroglobulin antibodies are present in 12–30% of patients with Graves' disease and 35–60% of patients with autoimmune hypothyroidism. They generally add little to the information obtained from the measurement of anti-thyroid peroxidase antibodies in diagnosing autoimmune hypothyroidism, although newer assays have been reported to be as sensitive as anti-thyroid peroxidase assays. The results of anti-thyroid peroxidase and anti-thyroglobulin antibody tests can differ in areas of iodine deficiency.

Anti-thyroglobulin antibodies interfere with measurements of thyroglobulin, and should be assayed in patients with differentiated thyroid cancer in whom serial thyroglobulin measurements are planned.

Anti-TSH-receptor antibodies are detectable in 70–100% of patients with Graves' disease (depending on the assay) and up to 20% of patients with autoimmune hypothyroidism (blocking antibodies). Measurement of stimulatory anti-TSH-receptor antibodies, which are themselves the cause of the hyperthyroidism, is the most sensitive antibody test for Graves' disease. An anti-TSH-receptor antibody test may also help to determine the cause of hyperthyroidism in pregnancy. Antibody presence in hypothyroidism may indicate reversible disease as the blocking antibody disappears. However, the assay is technically demanding and expensive. It is not routinely available in the UK.

Thyroglobulin is a tumor marker for differentiated thyroid cancer (see Chapter 7). Detectable levels also indicate the presence of endogenous thyroid activity in congenital hypothyroidism, while low thyroglobulin levels may reveal factitious hyperthyroidism (caused by undeclared thyroxine ingestion) in hyperthyroid individuals with low radio-iodine uptake.

Perchlorate discharge test. This test assesses the incorporation of iodine into thyroid hormone, which is abnormal in patients with autoimmune thyroiditis, hyperthyroidism, Pendred's syndrome or thyroid peroxidase defects. The test is now seldom performed except in specialized centers.

Thyroid imaging

Thyroid imaging is valuable in nodular disease or large goiters, but is not usually required in hypothyroid patients.

Radionuclide scans. The differential diagnosis of hyperthyroidism often requires measurement of the radioisotope uptake, commonly in conjunction with radionuclide imaging, which shows active tissue.

- ^{123}I scans are performed 24 hours after oral administration. This pure gamma emitter causes no thyroid damage and is the isotope of choice for 'hot' nodules (autonomously functioning thyroid adenomas with an enhanced ability to accumulate radio-iodine) and for most radio-iodine scanning.
- ^{99}Tc scans are performed 20 minutes after intravenous administration of the isotope. Although this is a more convenient test, it does not reliably distinguish 'hot' from 'cold' nodules.
- ^{131}I scans have largely been replaced by ^{123}I or ^{99}Tc scans, except in patients with thyroid cancer, particularly after large therapeutic doses of ^{131}I.

Radionuclide scans can distinguish Graves' disease from transient (destructive) thyroiditis by the difference in radio-iodine uptake – diffuse uptake in the former, but lack of uptake in the latter (see Figure 3.1, page 43). Radionuclide scans can also distinguish Graves' disease from a solitary toxic nodule or a toxic multinodular thyroid (see Figures 7.1 and 7.3, pages 111 and 117 respectively).

Although radioisotope scanning is useful in the follow-up of thyroid cancer, it is of limited value for investigating suspicious thyroid nodules, for which fine-needle aspiration is the investigation of choice. However, an ^{123}I scan should be performed to exclude a 'hot' nodule when serum TSH is below normal in association with a palpable or sizeable nodule (see Chapter 7).

Ultrasonography is a non-invasive, sensitive method of detecting thyroid cysts and nodules. It can be used to monitor changes in nodule size, although small, non-palpable nodules are seldom clinically significant (see Chapter 7). Newer ultrasound techniques may also identify those incidentally discovered smaller nodules that require additional testing. Ultrasonography is appropriate for screening patients with a history of head and neck irradiation, particularly in childhood, and is useful for postoperative follow-up of patients with thyroid carcinoma. It is rarely indicated in the investigation of hyperthyroidism or hypothyroidism, except possibly for amiodarone-induced hyperthyroidism.

Computed tomography and magnetic resonance imaging add little to ultrasonography in identifying thyroid nodules, but can be very useful in assessing retrosternal extension and compression of other structures, for example the trachea, in patients with large goiters, and for assessing infiltration of surrounding tissue in patients with malignant disease.

Key points – thyroid physiology and function tests

- The thyroid is the main site of iodine uptake in the body, incorporating it into the thyroid hormones T4 and T3.
- Most T3 (the active form of thyroid hormone) is produced by deiodination of T4 in the peripheral tissues.
- T4 and T3 production is controlled by a negative feedback mechanism involving the secretion of thyrotropin-releasing hormone by the hypothalamus and primarily thyroid-stimulating hormone (TSH) by the pituitary gland.
- The recommended daily intake of iodine for adults for normal production of thyroid hormone is 150–300 μg.
- The main thyroid function tests are TSH level (the most common first-line test), T4 or free T4 level and (usually for hyperthyroidism only) T3 or free T3 level.
- Thyroid imaging is valuable in nodular disease or large goiters, but is seldom required in hypothyroid patients.

Key references

Dayan CM. Interpretation of thyroid function tests. *Lancet* 2001;357: 619–24.

Haddow JE, Palomaki GE, Allan WC et al. Maternal thyroid deficiency during pregnancy and subsequent neuropsychological development of the child. *N Engl J Med* 1999;341: 549–55.

Ladenson PW, Singer PA, Ain KB et al. American Thyroid Association guidelines for detection of thyroid dysfunction. *Arch Intern Med* 2000;160:1573–5.

National Association of Clinical Biochemists. *Laboratory Medicine Practice Guidelines: Laboratory Support for the Diagnosis and Monitoring of Thyroid Disease.* 2002. http://www.nacb.org/lmpg/ thyroid_LMPG_PDF.stm (also published as Baloch Z, Carayon P, Conte-Devolx B et al. Laboratory medicine practice guidelines. Laboratory support for the diagnosis and monitoring of thyroid disease. *Thyroid* 2003;13:3–126).

Ross DS. Serum thyroid-stimulating hormone measurement for assessment of thyroid function and disease. *Endocrinol Metab Clin North Am* 2001;30:245–64.

Saravanan P, Dayan CM. Thyroid autoantibodies. *Endocrinol Metab Clin North Am* 2001;30:315–37.

Surks MI, Sievert R. Drugs and thyroid function. *N Engl J Med* 1995;333:1688–94.

Epidemiology

Clinical hyperthyroidism, defined as low thyroid-stimulating hormone (TSH) and raised T4, occurs in 0.5% of both the US and UK populations, while subclinical hyperthyroidism (TSH < 0.1 mU/L, T4 in the normal range) occurs in a further 0.7%. An additional 2.5% of women and 0.6% of men may have a previous history of hyperthyroidism. TSH values just below the normal range often revert to normal on repeat testing. Thyrotoxicosis can occur at any age in the adult population (Figure 2.1). Although the risk of developing hyperthyroidism increases two- to fourfold with age, this is a less dramatic increase than that of hypothyroidism with age (five- to tenfold) – 10–20% of women over the age of 65 have subclinical hypothyroidism. Prevalence estimates for hyperthyroidism in the elderly population are about 4% for women and 1.5% for men.

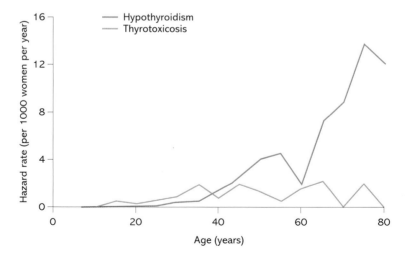

Figure 2.1 Risk for women of developing overt thyrotoxicosis (and hypothyroidism) at different ages. Redrawn with permission from Vanderpump MP et al. *Clin Endocrinol (Oxf)* 1995;43:55–68.

Of patients with clinical thyrotoxicosis referred to endocrine clinics:
- 65% have Graves' disease
- 20% have toxic multinodular goiter
- 5% have a solitary toxic nodule
- the remaining 10% have transient thyroiditis or an unclear etiology.

In areas of low iodine intake, the proportion of patients with toxic multinodular goiter is higher. Graves' disease can occur at any age, although it is rare in childhood; it is 7–10 times more common in women. Toxic nodular disease is uncommon in patients under 40 years old and probably accounts for much of the increasing prevalence of hyperthyroidism with age. It is likely that many cases of hyperthyroidism that occur because of the spontaneous resolution of thyroiditis go undiagnosed.

Etiology

The main causes of hyperthyroidism are summarized in Table 2.1, and are discussed in greater depth below. Measurement of radio-iodine uptake and a scan of radio-iodine distribution are very useful in the differential diagnosis of hyperthyroidism (see Chapter 3).

Graves' disease, also known as von Basedow's disease or diffuse toxic goiter, is an autoimmune condition in which anti-TSH-receptor antibodies stimulate the thyroid, hence the alternative name of thyroid-stimulating antibodies. Modern, sensitive assays are positive for these antibodies in more than 90% of cases, particularly in more severe cases of hyperthyroidism. Up to 70% of patients with Graves' disease have clinical or subclinical ophthalmopathy (see pages 32–34), which may occur because of low levels of TSH receptor expressed in the retro-orbital fibroblasts. Although the mechanism remains unclear, it appears that stressful life events are common in the 1–2 years preceding the onset of Graves' disease. Marked increases in the incidence of the disease have been reported in communities at war, for example a fivefold increase occurred during the civil war in the former Yugoslavia.

Toxic nodular disease. Most low TSH values in elderly patients are believed to be caused by nodular disease (see Chapter 7).

TABLE 2.1

Etiology of hyperthyroidism

Exogenous hormone*
Intentional or inadvertent suppressive treatment with T4 or T3
Factitious self-administration

Autonomous thyroid hormone production
Toxic adenoma[†]
Toxic multinodular goiter[†]
Struma ovarii (ectopic thyroid tissue in an ovarian dermoid tumor)[‡]
Thyroid cancer[‡]
Germline-activating TSH-receptor mutation[‡]

Thyroid stimulator present
Thyroid-stimulating antibody (Graves' disease)
HCG (normal pregnancy or hyperemesis gravidarum)
HCG (hydatidiform mole) or choriocarcinoma[‡]
TSH (TSH-secreting pituitary tumor)[‡]
TSH ('partial' pituitary resistance to thyroid hormone)[‡]

Excess release (destructive thyroiditis)
Painful postviral subacute thyroiditis
Painless subacute lymphocytic thyroiditis
(silent, postpartum, lithium-associated, cytokine-induced)
Amiodarone-induced destructive thyroiditis
Palpation thyroiditis[‡]
Thyroiditis after radiation[‡]
Malignant pseudothyroiditis[‡]
Pneumocystis thyroiditis[‡]

*Low serum thyroglobulin levels.
[†]May be precipitated by excess iodine.
[‡]Rare cause of hyperthyroidism.
HCG, human chorionic gonadotropin.

Other causes of hyperthyroidism. In addition to the common conditions

discussed above and the inadvertent or deliberate ingestion of excess thyroid hormone, hyperthyroidism may occur as result of a number of less common causes.

Human chorionic gonadotropin (HCG) can sometimes reach very high levels during pregnancy or in pregnancy-related states (e.g. hydatidiform mole) (see Chapter 6). In these situations, the HCG stimulates the thyroid by cross-reaction with TSH at the TSH receptor.

Iodine-induced thyrotoxicosis. The effects of iodine on the thyroid gland are complex. While chronic iodine deficiency predisposes patients to hypothyroidism and may stimulate the growth of thyroid nodules, pharmacological doses of iodine in, for example, amiodarone or iodine-containing contrast media can induce thyrotoxicosis in autonomous nodular thyroid glands.

Destructive thyroiditis. Several conditions cause subacute destructive inflammation in the thyroid (see Table 2.1), leading to the discharge of stored hormone. The result is transient hyperthyroidism, lasting 1–3 months, which resolves when the previously stored thyroid hormone is depleted. During this period of hyperthyroidism, no thyroid hormone synthesis occurs and thionamide therapy is ineffective. Hyperthyroidism is often followed by a similar or longer duration of hypothyroidism, before returning spontaneously to euthyroidism.

A relatively common cause of destructive thyroiditis is postviral subacute (de Quervain's) thyroiditis, which is associated with a painful, markedly tender thyroid (often confused with a 'sore throat'), fever and a raised erythrocyte sedimentation rate.

Lymphocytic subacute thyroiditis and its postpartum variant are painless and are often both classified as painless subacute thyroiditis. Silent (painless lymphocytic subacute) and postpartum thyroiditis often recur, but postviral thyroiditis usually does not. Painless lymphocytic thyroiditis is increasingly being reported in patients:

- receiving interferon α therapy for viral hepatitis
- receiving bone marrow transplantation (particularly patients with graft-versus-host disease)
- receiving interleukin therapy for malignancy
- recovering from T-cell-depleting therapy.

These treatments have also been associated with true Graves' disease and hypothyroidism.

Type 2 amiodarone-induced thyrotoxicosis (see below) is a form of destructive thyroiditis.

Amiodarone-induced thyrotoxicosis. Amiodarone is an iodinated antiarrhythmic and antianginal drug that can induce both hypothyroidism and hyperthyroidism. Amiodarone-induced hyperthyroidism may occur at any time after the start of amiodarone therapy or up to 1 year after it has been discontinued. It is much more common in iodine-deficient areas, where the incidence approaches 10% of amiodarone-treated patients. Type 1 amiodarone-induced thyrotoxicosis may develop in patients with pre-existing nodular thyroid glands or with potential Graves' disease; it can be very severe, and is due to the high iodine content of amiodarone. Type 2 amiodarone-induced thyrotoxicosis is more common and, although it is self-limiting, it can be severe and cause cardiac decompensation if it is not treated promptly; it is a form of destructive thyroiditis caused by direct toxicity of amiodarone or its metabolites.

TSH-induced hyperthyroidism (central hyperthyroidism) is a very rare form of thyrotoxicosis caused by a TSH-secreting pituitary tumor. It can be missed in routine thyroid function tests, as TSH levels are often in the 'normal' range; for this reason, when hyperthyroidism is suspected, T4 or free T4 and/or T3 or free T3 (which will be elevated) should be measured in addition to TSH to diagnose this condition.

Germline-activating TSH-receptor mutations are a rare cause of congenital hyperthyroidism, which characteristically recurs after thyroidectomy.

Subclinical hyperthyroidism

Subclinical hyperthyroidism is characterized by a suppressed serum TSH with serum levels of thyroid hormones still in the reference range. TSH levels below 0.1 mU/L occur in 1–2% of the adult population not receiving thyroid hormone, and in 3% of individuals over 80 years old. Subnormal TSH values of 0.1 mU/L or above are even more common. Patients receiving supraphysiological doses of T4 are commonly found to have a subnormal serum TSH concentration, known as exogenous subclinical hyperthyroidism. When TSH suppression is not the goal of such therapy, the T4 dose should be decreased. A persistently low TSH level that is not due to excess T4 administration, non-thyroidal illness or other drugs is called endogenous subclinical hyperthyroidism.

A TSH concentration below 0.1 mU/L is associated with a 30% 10-year risk of atrial fibrillation (a threefold increased risk) in patients over 60 years old, and a twofold increase in mortality from circulatory diseases over 10 years. In estrogen-deficient (particularly postmenopausal) women, subclinical hyperthyroidism is associated with decreased bone density. Other possible consequences include left ventricular hypertrophy. The risk of progression to overt hyperthyroidism appears to be low, at about 1–2% per year.

Clinical presentation

The clinical features of hyperthyroidism, which often resemble those associated with an anxiety state, are summarized in Table 2.2. Agitation, irritability, anxiety, sleeplessness and emotional lability may dominate the clinical picture, though an apathetic (withdrawn) presentation of hyperthyroidism is also occasionally seen. Absolute levels of T4 or T3 often correlate poorly with the severity of symptoms in an individual patient; the thyroid in Graves' disease is often only minimally enlarged or even normal in size, despite marked thyrotoxicosis (Figure 2.2). Respiratory (diaphragmatic) muscle weakness, increased hypoxic respiratory drive and cardiac failure can all contribute to dyspnea in thyrotoxicosis.

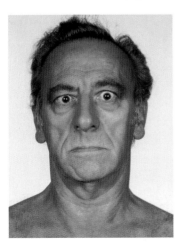

Figure 2.2 Man with Graves' disease presenting with mild thyroid eye disease. Other clinical features included weight loss, 'hyperactive' appearance and small goiter.

TABLE 2.2

Clinical features of hyperthyroidism

Common features	Uncommon features
• Weight loss with good appetite	• Urticaria, itching
• Heat intolerance	• Weight gain (marked increase in appetite)
• Palpitations	• Ankle edema without heart failure
• Anxiety	
• Dyspnea	• Heart failure
• Irritability	• Isolated persistent vomiting
• Sweating	• Oligomenorrhea/amenorrhea
• General eye symptoms (i.e. lid retraction, lid lag)	• Anemia
	• Hypercalcemia
• Exophthalmos and inflammatory eye signs*	• Fever of unknown origin
	• Unexplained osteoporosis
• Hyperdefecation (particularly in the morning)	• Gynecomastia
• Raised alkaline phosphatase	• Bulbar myopathy
• Tremor	• 'Apathetic thyrotoxicosis', including decreased appetite, constipation and absence of tachycardia
• Proximal myopathy	
• Atrial fibrillation	
• Thyroid bruit*	• Pretibial myxedema*
	• Acropachy*

*Only found in Graves' disease; not caused by hyperthyroidism per se.

Ophthalmic features. Lid retraction and lid lag can occur with any cause of thyrotoxicosis, and simply reflect increased activity of the levator palpebrae muscles. True thyroid eye disease – with exophthalmos and inflammatory eye signs – is diagnostic of Graves' disease (Figure 2.3).

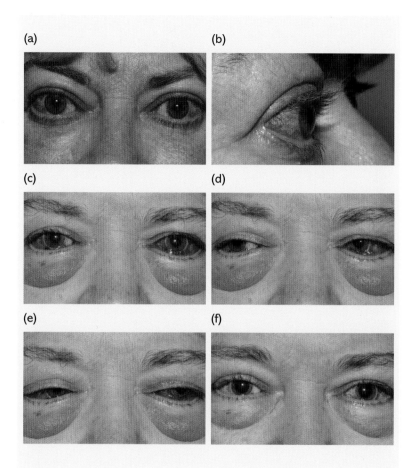

Figure 2.3 True thyroid eye disease, with inflammatory eye signs in 2 patients with Graves' disease: (a) and (b) Active thyroid eye disease with marked supraorbital edema and some redness of the eyes. (c) Marked infraorbital edema and chemosis (conjunctival edema), especially of the left eye. (d) and (e) Restricted eye movements when the patient is asked to look right (d) and then left (e); the patient also had optic nerve compression. (f) After significant reduction of disease activity with immunosuppression; the eyes are now white and eye movements fully recovered. Note: proptosis is not present in either of these patients, emphasising that each manifestation of thyroid eye disease (proptosis, soft-tissue swelling, restricted eye movements and optic nerve compression) can occur independently of the others.

TABLE 2.3

Key features of thyroid eye disease using the NOSPECS* mnemonic

Signs	Comment
N No eye signs or symptoms	
O Only signs of hyperthyroidism	Lid lag, lid retraction
S Soft-tissue swelling	Periorbital edema; red, itchy eye
P Proptosis (exophthalmos)	
E Extraocular muscle involvement	Often results in diplopia; pain, especially on upgaze
C Corneal involvement	Generally a consequence of severe proptosis with failure to protect the cornea
S Sight loss due to compressive optic neuropathy	REFER URGENTLY to an ophthalmologist skilled in Graves' disease

*The 'SPECS' elements of the mnemonic are specific for Graves' disease and are not found in other forms of hyperthyroidism.

Each of the key features of thyroid eye disease (Tables 2.3 and 2.4) can occur independently of the others. Common early symptoms are often missed by clinicians; they include 'grittiness', redness or watering of one or both eyes, often with photophobia and swelling around the eyes, particularly early in the morning. Patient complaints of impaired vision may be related to:

- increased secretions (improved with frequent blinking)
- diplopia (normal vision in each eye independently)
- optic neuropathy.

The earliest signs of optic nerve compression are color desaturation (e.g. on Ishihara color charts), altitudinal field defects and, at a later stage, a decline in visual acuity. Compression of the optic nerve requires urgent referral to an ophthalmologist with special expertise in this area.

Other clinical features. Pretibial myxedema, a non-pitting, disfiguring skin infiltration that generally involves the anterior tibial region and

TABLE 2.4

Clinically important aspects of thyroid eye disease

- Proptosis is not always present
- Often asymmetrical; 10–15% unilateral
- Occurs before or after thyrotoxicosis in up to 50% of cases
- Occurs without thyrotoxicosis in 10% of cases
- Very occasionally associated with Hashimoto's thyroiditis with hypothyroidism
- Can improve spontaneously
- Not necessarily helped by treatment of thyrotoxicosis
- May be exacerbated by radio-iodine
- Smoking is the major risk factor for high-grade ophthalmopathy
- Psychological effects should not be underestimated
- May be worsened by periods of hypothyroidism

dorsum of the foot, and thyroid acropachy (or 'clubbing'), caused by proliferation of the distal soft tissues, especially the nail beds, which results in thickening and widening of the digital extremeties, are uncommon manifestations of Graves' disease that tend to occur (almost always) in patients who also have thyroid eye disease (Figure 2.4).

A thyroid bruit – the sound of increased blood flow through the thyroid – is a useful finding, as it is virtually diagnostic of Graves' disease and excludes destructive thyroiditis.

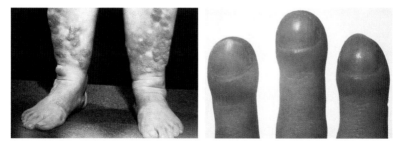

Figure 2.4 Uncommon manifestations of Graves' disease: (a) pretibial myxedema, and (b) thyroid acropachy ('clubbing').

Weight loss alone or atrial fibrillation alone is common in elderly patients with hyperthyroidism. Weight loss with decreased appetite, constipation and absent tachycardia are confusing clinical features that can create a suspicion of malignancy. Isolated vomiting is a rare but recognized presentation.

In children, hyperthyroidism is almost always due to Graves' disease and is more resistant to drug-induced remission.

Spontaneous remissions occur in 10–30% of untreated or β-blocker-treated patients with Graves' disease. Nevertheless, it is unwise to wait for a remission when hyperthyroidism is persistent or symptomatic. Hyperthyroidism due to toxic adenoma or toxic multinodular goiter seldom improves spontaneously.

Biochemical consequences of thyrotoxicosis

Hormonal increases. Sex-hormone-binding globulin (SHBG) increases in hyperthyroidism and can be a useful marker of thyroid hormone action. In men with hyperthyroidism, increases in SHBG result in a marked elevation of serum testosterone and estradiol.

Hematologic abnormalities

Anemia. Microcytic, normocytic or macrocytic anemia occurs in 10–25% of thyrotoxic patients. The anemia is usually mild, and may result from ineffective erythropoiesis and coincident deficiencies in iron, vitamin B_{12} or folate.

Mild granulocytopenia may occur in a minority of patients with Graves' disease, as a result of thyroid-stimulating antibodies binding to TSH receptors in granulocytes and inducing a mild immune neutropenia.

Alkaline phosphatase and liver aminotransferases are raised in about 65% and 30% of patients, respectively, at presentation. These benign enzymatic changes may be difficult to distinguish from hepatitis induced by anti-thyroid drugs if baseline values are not recorded. At baseline the elevated alkaline phosphatase originates from both liver and bone. After therapy, alkaline phosphatase originating from bone rises further in most patients; these elevations may persist for up to 1 year.

Complications of hyperthyroidism

Atrial fibrillation. Patients treated for thyrotoxicosis experience excess mortality from cardiovascular and cerebrovascular disease, especially in the first year. Although the reason for this is unclear, atrial fibrillation occurs in 5–15% of patients with hyperthyroidism. The incidence of atrial fibrillation increases with age, and is associated with an increased risk of stroke.

After treatment of thyrotoxicosis, 60–70% of patients revert to sinus rhythm within 12 weeks of achieving euthyroidism; spontaneous reversion is unusual after this time. Patients with hyperthyroidism and atrial fibrillation (especially the elderly and those with heart disease) should therefore be considered for anticoagulation treatment and electrical cardioversion if sinus rhythm is not re-established within 3 months of achieving euthyroidism. Higher than usual doses of digoxin are required to control the heart rate during hyperthyroid atrial fibrillation, and β-blockers are recommended as first-line therapy.

Osteoporosis. Thyroid hormone has direct effects on bone resorption and increases bone turnover. Consequences include occasional hypercalcemia, reduced bone mineral density (particularly of cortical bone), hypercalciuria and, occasionally, formation of renal stones. The fracture rate may increase slightly before and immediately after diagnosis, but this does not appear to be sustained. Muscle weakness and impaired judgment can contribute to falls, increasing the risk.

Treatment allows bone density to recover, but not always to pre-existing levels; important bone structural elements may be irreversibly damaged. Fracture rate may return to normal more rapidly after surgical treatment than after radio-iodine therapy, perhaps indicating that a rapid return to euthyroidism is beneficial for the skeleton.

Thyrotoxic storm is a rare condition characterized by:
- severe hyperthyroidism associated with fever
- disproportionate tachycardia
- central nervous system dysfunction (especially confusion or severe irritability)
- gastrointestinal dysfunction (diarrhea, vomiting, jaundice).

Old literature sources report mortality as 10–75%; this rate is likely to have changed, but because of the rarity of the condition no recent series have been reported. Levels of thyroid hormones are high, but no different from levels in many individuals without a crisis. Thyrotoxic storm is often precipitated by intercurrent infection, but can also occur in conjunction with other illnesses, with thyroid and other surgery in untreated thyrotoxic patients, and after radio-iodine therapy or trauma to the thyroid gland.

Periodic paralysis. Hypokalemic periodic paralysis is a rare manifestation of Graves' disease that occurs mostly, but not exclusively, in men of Oriental descent, and is characterized by episodes of leg, arm or (uncommonly) respiratory weakness. Treatment focuses on the rapid correction of thyrotoxicosis and any hypokalemia.

Thyroid eye disease, also known as Graves' ophthalmopathy, dysthyroid eye disease or thyroid-associated ophthalmopathy, is clinically detectable in 10–20% of patients with Graves' disease and is severe in 5% (see Figure 2.3). Sensitive techniques, such as orbital ultrasonography, computed tomography and magnetic resonance imaging, show its presence in 50–70% of patients. Thyroid eye disease is more common than expected in men and smokers when compared with the general prevalence of Graves' hyperthyroidism in these groups. Thyroid eye disease commonly develops over 3–6 months and then remains stable for at least 1 year in 80–90% of cases, continuing to progress in 10–15%. Symptoms may continue for many years. The first appearance of thyroid eye disease may be separated from hyperthyroidism by months or years, presenting either before or after the change in thyroid function. Eye disease that precedes thyroid dysfunction can cause particular diagnostic confusion.

Thyroid eye disease tends to worsen more often after radio-iodine therapy than after thionamide treatment or thyroidectomy, particularly in patients with pre-existing eye disease. However, the deleterious effects of smoking and possibly of hypothyroidism on thyroid eye disease may have confounded the results of the controlled trials on the effect of radio-iodine alone.

Key points – hyperthyroidism: etiology and presentation

- Clinical hyperthyroidism is defined as low levels of thyroid-stimulating hormone (TSH) and raised thyroid hormone (T4 and T3).
- The majority of cases of clinical thyrotoxicosis are due to Graves' disease (an autoimmune condition in which anti-TSH-receptor antibodies stimulate the thyroid); other common causes are multinodular goiter and toxic adenoma.
- Amiodarone-induced hyperthyroidism may be due to iodine-induced thyrotoxicosis (multinodular goiter or Graves' disease) or destructive thyroiditis.
- A radio-iodine uptake and scan is important to distinguish the various causes of hyperthyroidism, and to diagnose transient hyperthyroidism due to destructive thyroiditis.
- Subclinical hyperthyroidism is characterized by a suppressed serum TSH with serum levels of thyroid hormones still in the reference range.
- The clinical features of hyperthyroidism may include irritability, anxiety, sleeplessness and emotional lability.
- Lid retraction and lid lag can occur with any cause of thyrotoxicosis, but true thyroid eye disease (with exophthalmos and inflammatory eye signs) is a clinical feature of Graves' disease.
- Possible complications of hyperthyroidism include atrial fibrillation, osteoporosis, thyrotoxic storm (rare) and periodic paralysis (rare).

Thyroid eye disease remains the most difficult aspect of Graves' disease to manage. The autoimmune process is believed to be a cross-reaction between thyroid autoantibodies and thyroid-type proteins expressed in the retro-orbital adipose tissue, including the TSH receptor. This ultimately results in edema in the extraocular muscles and retro-orbital space, which in turn causes orbital protrusion

39

(proptosis). Over time, lymphocytic infiltration, inflammation and swelling give way to fibrosis, and the disease changes from an active or 'wet' phase, responsive to immunosuppression, to a 'dry' fibrotic phase, in which only corrective surgery is effective (see page 63).

Pretibial myxedema (dermopathy). This rare complication of Graves' disease occurs almost exclusively (97%) in patients who also have thyroid eye disease. Pretibial myxedema appears as a non-pitting, disfiguring skin infiltration that generally involves the anterior tibial region and dorsum of the foot (see Figure 2.4a), and very occasionally involves the arm. Therapy includes topical glucocorticoid administration under plastic occlusion, but is generally unsatisfactory.

Clubbing (thyroid acropachy) is quite rare (see Figure 2.4b).

Key references

Bjoro T, Holmen J, Kruger O et al. Prevalence of thyroid disease, thyroid dysfunction and thyroid peroxidase antibodies in a large, unselected population. The Health Study of Nord-Trondelag (HUNT). *Eur J Endocrinol* 2000;143:639–47.

Cooper DS. Hyperthyroidism. *Lancet* 2003;362:459–68.

Hollowell JG, Staehling NW, Flanders WD et al. Serum TSH, T(4), and thyroid antibodies in the United States population (1988 to 1994): National Health and Nutrition Examination Survey (NHANES III). *J Clin Endocrinol Metab* 2002;87:489–99.

Schwartz KM, Fatourechi V, Ahmed DD, Pond GR. Dermopathy of Graves' disease (pretibial myxedema): long-term outcome. *J Clin Endocrinol Metab* 2002;87:438–46.

Toft AD. Clinical practice. Subclinical hyperthyroidism. *N Engl J Med* 2001;345:512–16.

Vestergaard P, Moskilde L. Fractures in patients with hyperthyroidism and hypothyroidism: a nationwide follow-up study in 16,249 patients. *Thyroid* 2002;12:411–19.

Diagnosis

Biochemical confirmation. When hyperthyroidism is clinically suspected, the combination of undetectable TSH and raised T4/free T4 or T3 is usually present, making biochemical confirmation straightforward. If the T4 or free T4 levels are not raised, T3 estimation should be performed, because in some cases only T3 is above the normal range (T3 toxicosis). The combination of a normal free T4, T3 or free T3 and a suppressed TSH is called subclinical hyperthyroidism, which is the earliest stage of hyperthyroidism (see Chapter 2). If TSH is in the normal range, but hyperthyroidism is suspected on clinical grounds, T4, free T3 and T3 should be measured to exclude interference with the TSH assay or a rare condition such as a TSH-secreting pituitary tumor or pituitary resistance to thyroid hormone.

Differential diagnosis. In most instances of hyperthyroidism, measuring 24-hour radio-iodine uptake and a radionuclide scan will indicate the type of hyperthyroidism present (Tables 3.1 and 3.2). Despite the useful application of radionuclide scanning, many endocrinologists, particularly in the UK, do not routinely perform the procedure in hyperthyroid patients. Instead, they take a pragmatic approach, in which scanning is reserved for patients with postpartum disease, a short history of thyrotoxicosis and a high index of suspicion for destructive thyroiditis, or for complex cases. Some of the differential diagnoses detailed below indicate the usefulness of radionuclide scanning, which is routinely employed in the USA.

Graves' disease. Diffuse uptake on radionuclide scanning is virtually diagnostic of Graves' disease, even when the overall uptake is within normal limits (Figure 3.1).

Anti-TSH-receptor antibodies are the most specific test for Graves' disease, but they may be absent in 5–10% of cases, especially in mild disease, and the test is often not routinely available.

TABLE 3.1

Hyperthyroidism with increased or normal radio-iodine uptake

Diagnosis	Distribution of radio-iodine uptake*
Graves' disease	Diffuse uptake, although overall uptake may be in the reference range (see Figure 3.1)
Toxic multinodular goiter	Irregular uptake or multiple hot nodules (see Figure 7.3); overall uptake in large glands may be very low
Solitary hot nodule	Uptake into single nodule only (see Figure 7.1)
TSH-induced or HCG-induced hyperthyroidism	Diffuse uptake

*Similar results obtained with ^{99}Tc scanning.
HCG, human chorionic gonadotropin.

TABLE 3.2

Hyperthyroidism with near-nil 24-hour radio-iodine uptake in the neck

Diagnosis	Comment
Exogenous thyroid hormone ingestion (including factitious)	Low serum thyroglobulin
Destructive thyroiditis – painful postviral subacute thyroiditis – painless lymphocytic subacute thyroiditis – amiodarone-induced destructive thyrotoxicosis (type 2) and others	Transient hyperthyroidism (includes postpartum thyroiditis); often followed by hypothyroidism; painful neck in postviral form
Struma ovarii (ectopic thyroid tissue)	Uptake over pelvis but not in neck
Excess iodine administration in conjunction with causes of hyperthyroidism (see Table 3.1), e.g. a CT scan with contrast performed just before a radio-iodine uptake test	

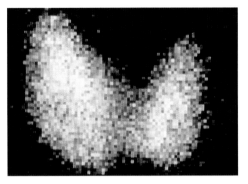

Figure 3.1 Diffuse thyroid uptake of iodine in Graves' disease.

Measurement of anti-TSH-receptor antibodies is generally unnecessary if a radionuclide scan is obtained, but is most helpful when a radionuclide scan cannot be carried out, for example during pregnancy or nursing, or because of patient preference.

Hot nodule. This is defined as a nodular region of the thyroid gland that takes up large amounts of radio-iodine, hence it is visualized as a 'hot spot' on the thyroid scan and can be diagnosed as a single toxic nodule (see Figure 7.1).

Toxic multinodular goiter is indicated by irregular uptake or multiple hot areas on radionuclide scanning (see Figure 7.3).

Destructive thyroiditis is suggested when radio-iodine uptake over 24 hours or during radionuclide scanning is absent. This condition should also be suspected if there is a very short history of hyperthyroidism (4–6 weeks or less), if it spontaneously improves over 4–6 weeks, or if it rapidly progresses to hypothyroidism.

The three common types of destructive thyroiditis are:

- painful postviral subacute thyroiditis
- painless lymphocytic subacute thyroiditis
- amiodarone-induced destructive thyrotoxicosis (type 2).

Painful postviral subacute thyroiditis can be suspected from the exquisitely tender thyroid. The erythrocyte sedimentation rate is markedly elevated, often over 100.

Painless lymphocytic subacute thyroiditis and postpartum thyroiditis must be identified to avoid unnecessary treatment being given for these conditions. In addition, if the clinician suspects undisclosed thyroxine ingestion, painless lymphocytic thyroiditis must be distinguished from

43

factitious hyperthyroidism – although both have a low 24-hour radio-iodine uptake, serum thyroglobulin is uniquely low in factitious hyperthyroidism in contrast to all other types of hyperthyroidism with a low radio-iodine uptake.

Amiodarone-induced thyrotoxicosis. Distinguishing between type 1 and type 2 amiodarone-induced thyrotoxicosis can be difficult (see page 30). Color-flow Doppler ultrasonography reveals normal-to-increased thyroid blood flow in type 1 disease, whereas it is markedly reduced in type 2 disease. Unfortunately, this test gives uncertain results in 20% or more of patients. Radio-iodine uptake is often low even in iodine-induced disease, because of excess iodine release from the amiodarone. A therapeutic response to glucocorticoid therapy may be the most reliable 'test' for amiodarone-induced destructive thyrotoxicosis.

Thyroid eye disease is generally a straightforward diagnosis when hyperthyroidism is present, although low-grade disease with soft-tissue signs only can often be overlooked (see pages 32–35). In euthyroid patients, the presence of anti-thyroid peroxidase or thyroid-stimulating antibodies is helpful but not always seen. Magnetic resonance imaging (MRI) or computed tomography of the orbit, demonstrating typical eye muscle changes, is useful for confirming the diagnosis, and MRI can also help to determine disease activity.

Choice of treatment

Three standard treatments are available for hyperthyroidism that is not due to destructive thyroiditis:

- thionamide drugs
- radio-iodine (^{131}I)
- surgery.

Specific aspects of each treatment are discussed in detail in later sections. As all three treatments are effective, patients often ask for guidance as to which to choose. Table 3.3 (pages 46–47) summarizes the advantages and disadvantages in a patient-friendly form. Comparison of all three treatments in a single study showed little difference in final outcome or patient acceptability, although surgery achieved the quickest return to euthyroidism (Figure 3.2).

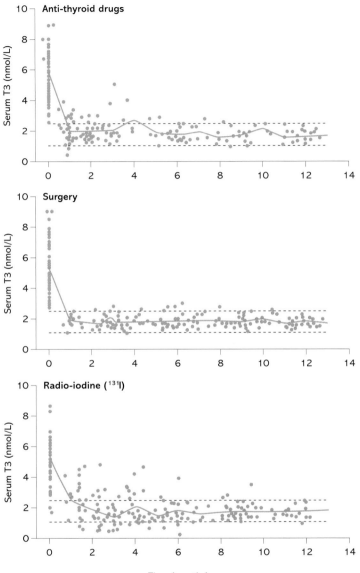

Figure 3.2 Thyroid function following thionamide therapy, radio-iodine or surgery in a randomized controlled trial. Individual (dots) and mean (blue line) values for serum T3 are shown for each treatment. Redrawn with permission from Torring O et al. Graves' hyperthyroidism: treatment with antithyroid drugs, surgery or radio-iodine. *J Clin Endocrinol Metab* 1996;81:2986–93. Copyright 1996, The Endocrine Society.

TABLE 3.3

Patient information sheet on different treatments for Graves' disease

Treatment	You cannot use it if...
Anti-thyroid drugs • carbimazole (methimazole) • propylthiouracil	You have had a severe reaction to one of these drugs
Radio-iodine	You are pregnant or breastfeeding Use with caution in patients with significant Graves' eye disease
Surgery	If your hyperthyroidism has not been controlled with medication before surgery (this can sometimes be just a β-blocker)

Anti-thyroid drug treatment blocks thyroid hormone production, is non-destructive and avoids exposure to radiation or surgery. Thionamides are thought to facilitate the disappearance of thyroid-stimulating antibodies, either by direct immunosuppressive effects or as a consequence of achieving the euthyroid state. A therapeutic course of thionamides may promote sustained remission in patients with Graves' disease, allowing some to stop all medication. However, thionamide treatment is only a temporary measure for multinodular goiter and

Advantages	Disadvantages
• Relatively fast effect (6–12 weeks) • Sudden swings in thyroid hormone level unlikely • Painless • Safe in sick patients	• 12–18-month course of tablets • Thyroid overactivity returns within 12 months in 40–50% of patients after treatment, and later in a further 25% • 5% risk of rash or minor side effects • 0.5% (1 in 200) risk of serious effects on white blood cells
• Painless • Permanent – low chance of overactivity returning	• Slow action (6 weeks to 6 months); may require medication over this period • 10–15% of people require repeat therapy • High chance of thyroid under-activity needing thyroxine tablets • May worsen eye problems • Thyroid may become underactive many years later
• Quick (effect within days) • Permanent – low chance of overactivity returning	• General anesthetic carries risks • 1% chance of damage to the nerve to the vocal cords (hoarse voice) or to calcium-controlling parathyroid glands • Discomfort/neck scar

toxic nodule, and these conditions will relapse when the treatment is stopped. Definitive therapy requires radio-iodine or surgery (see Chapter 7).

Radio-iodine therapy is painless and, despite the use of radiation, has an excellent long-term safety record. However, it may be slow to act and frequently results in long-term hypothyroidism. It is first-line treatment for hyperthyroidism in the USA and for many physicians in

47

other parts of the world. A survey in 1987 suggested that it was used as first-line treatment in Europe in 22% of cases. In the UK, it is used as first-line treatment in around 40% of patients.

Surgery. Although surgery can achieve prompt euthyroidism, most patients prefer to avoid this option. Surgeons usually require patients to be euthyroid before surgery, which means that a period of treatment with thionamides is still required.

Medical management

Symptomatic therapy. β-blockers effectively treat tachycardia, tremor, anxiety and heat intolerance, and they are useful for the early treatment of thyrotoxicosis, including the hyperthyroid phase of transient thyroiditis, thyrotoxic storm and uncontrolled atrial fibrillation. High-dose propranolol minimally inhibits T4-to-T3 conversion, but other β-blockers do not alter serum levels of thyroid hormones.

The hypothyroid phase of destructive thyroiditis should be treated with T4 if it is symptomatic or prolonged. Pain in viral subacute thyroiditis often responds to non-steroidal anti-inflammatory agents, but glucocorticoids are occasionally required. Glucocorticoid therapy is an important therapeutic option in amiodarone-induced thyrotoxicosis.

In selected cases of hyperthyroidism, thyroidectomy can be performed after the administration of very high doses of β-blockers.

Thionamides. Propylthiouracil and methimazole (prescribed in the USA) – or the prodrug form carbimazole (prescribed in the UK) – primarily inhibit the synthesis of thyroid hormones. In general, methimazole/ carbimazole is the first choice of drug. Its long half-life allows once-daily dosage (Table 3.4), the advantages of which are:
• improved compliance
• greater potency
• less potential for toxicity.

Propylthiouracil is reserved for use during pregnancy, patients who are intolerant of methimazole/carbimazole and possibly patients with thyrotoxic storm.

TABLE 3.4

Comparison of the advantages of the two most commonly used thionamide drugs, methimazole/carbimazole and propylthiouracil

Methimazole/Carbimazole	Propylthiouracil
• Single daily dose	• Possibly safer in pregnancy
• More potent	• Can be used in cases of mild methimazole/carbimazole intolerance
• High-dose tablets available, e.g. 20 mg carbimazole/ 10 mg methimazole	
• Increasing toxicity with long-term use not documented (compare appearance of ANCA positivity after years of PTU therapy)	

ANCA, anti-neutrophil cytoplasmic antibodies; PTU, propylthiouracil.

Dosage. For moderate or severe hyperthyroidism, typical starting doses are:
• 30 mg methimazole (40 mg carbimazole) once daily
• 300 mg propylthiouracil in three divided doses.

When hyperthyroidism is mild, lower initial doses may be given. Higher doses confer little benefit, may carry an increased risk of side effects and are generally reserved for severely ill patients. At the doses described here, about 85% of compliant patients will be euthyroid or hypothyroid in 4 weeks (Figure 3.3), although the response depends on the initial level of T4.

When thyroid function tests enter the normal range, the dose should be reduced (typically to 5–15 mg of methimazole/carbimazole) and titrated according to thyroid status, as indicated by 3-monthly thyroid function tests. A common error is to discontinue these drugs when early hypothyroidism develops, which almost invariably results in recurrent hyperthyroidism. Alternatively, the high dose can be maintained and thyroxine added (typically 100 μg of T4).

49

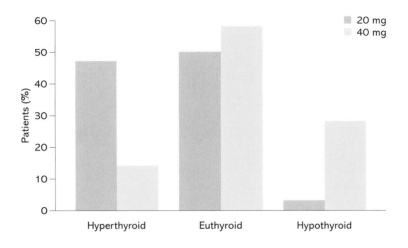

Figure 3.3 Thyroid status after 4 weeks of treatment with carbimazole. Adapted from Page SR et al. *Clin Endocrinol (Oxf)* 1996;45:511–16.

Although it is not used routinely, this 'block–replace' regimen has a number of advantages:

- it seldom requires dose adjustment
- it is straightforward
- it is particularly useful when close follow-up is difficult or when patients have previously suffered from alternating hyperthyroidism and hypothyroidism while on therapy.

The 'block–replace' regimen is not used in pregnancy, as high-dose thionamides cross the placenta more readily than the T4 replacement.

Duration. Treatment guidelines recommend an initial course of treatment lasting 6 months to 2 years; 18 months of treatment results in a higher remission rate than 6 months' treatment, but extending treatment to 42 months has no advantage. Many clinicians in the USA prescribe a 12-month course of therapy; an 18-month course of treatment is more common in the UK.

When treatment is stopped, patients are observed closely for relapse in the first year and then at 6–12-month intervals. Around 50–60% of patients with Graves' disease will still be euthyroid 1 year after treatment. Some patients who relapse refuse definitive therapy with radio-iodine or surgery; in the absence of allergic reactions, methimazole/carbimazole therapy may be continued indefinitely in these patients. It is less advisable to use propylthiouracil for long-term treatment, because the risk of associated vasculitis increases with duration of treatment.

Relapse is more common in:
- young people (often over 70% in children)
- men
- patients with large goiters (> 40 g or twice normal size)
- patients with high initial T3/T4 ratios (or T3 levels)
- patients who continue to test positive for anti-TSH-receptor antibodies.

None of these factors is robust enough, however, to guide clinical practice, although some endocrinologists continue treatment until the anti-TSH-receptor antibody titer becomes negative. It should be obvious that relapse is inevitable if thionamides cannot be tapered without recurrent hyperthyroidism.

Side effects of thionamide drugs (Table 3.5), particularly the risk of agranulocytosis, must be explained to patients. A standard advice card is useful (Figure 3.4).

TABLE 3.5

Side effects of thionamides

Major	Minor (about 5%)
• Agranulocytosis (0.2–0.5%)	• Rash, including urticaria
• Aplastic anemia	• Arthralgia (may be a warning sign of vasculitis)
• Hepatitis (with PTU)	
• Cholestatic jaundice (with methimazole or carbimazole)	• Fever
	• Transient granulocytopenia
• Vasculitis – ANCA positive, primarily with PTU	

ANCA, anti-neutrophil cytoplasmic antibodies; PTU, propylthiouracil.

Agranulocytosis usually occurs within the first weeks of treatment, although it can occur much later when starting a second course of the drug, and at relatively low doses. If it occurs early in therapy, alternative treatment (typically radio-iodine, possibly supported by other measures) should be planned immediately, as discontinuation of thionamides at this

---

Warning: PLEASE READ THIS NOW.
Carbimazole (methimazole) or PTU treatment and sore mouth/throat

You have been started on carbimazole (methimazole) or PTU treatment for an overactive thyroid. This is a very safe treatment that has been used for over 50 years.

However, very rarely, a patient reacts to the drug with a sudden loss of white blood cells ('granulocytes') from the blood. This results in a very high risk from infections and the drug **MUST BE STOPPED IMMEDIATELY**. The first sign of this happening is A SEVERE SORE MOUTH OR THROAT or mouth ulcerations FOR NO OBVIOUS REASON. Unexplained fever may also occur.

If you suspect this may have happened:
1. Do NOT take any more doses of the tablet.
2. Contact an emergency doctor or an emergency department THE SAME DAY (even if it is a weekend) and show this card or the tablets.

TO THE DOCTOR:

This patient is on CARBIMAZOLE (methimazole, PTU). If a sore throat or mouth is present it may indicate agranulocytosis, a very rare side effect of anti-thyroid drugs. Please:

1. Stop carbimazole (methimazole) or PTU immediately

2. Check granulocyte count urgently, NOT just the total white cell count (which may be normal because the lymphocytes are unaffected). If the granulocyte count is $< 1.0 \times 10^9$/L, do NOT recommence treatment, and treat patient for granulocytopenia. If level is $1.0–2.0 \times 10^9$/L, repeat granulocyte count the next day off anti-thyroid drugs. If level is $> 2.0 \times 10^9$/L, it is safe to continue treatment. Both carbimazole and thyrotoxicosis also cause a mild reduction in white cell count which is of no significance. A skin rash on carbimazole is also common and does not indicate granulocytopenia.

Figure 3.4 Warning card for patients starting thionamide therapy for hyperthyroidism.

stage can result in severe uncontrolled hyperthyroidism within 2–3 weeks. The risk of agranulocytosis in patients maintained for years on very low doses, for example 5 mg methimazole/carbimazole, appears to be minimal. Some endocrinologists are comfortable using low-dose methimazole/carbimazole (but not propylthiouracil) indefinitely in patients who have relapsed or in elderly patients with multinodular goiter who refuse radio-iodine treatment. The following aspects of thionamide-induced agranulocytosis are important.

- Prompt (same day) discontinuation of thionamides is critical – fatalities have occurred when this is delayed, but when discontinuation is prompt the granulocyte count recovers within 10–14 days (more rapidly if the initial count is at least 0.1×10^9/L). Administration of granulocyte colony-stimulating factor (G-CSF) shortens recovery time only in patients with a detectable initial count.
- The differential granulocyte count must be measured – the total white cell count may be within the normal range, as lymphocytes are not affected.
- Agranulocytosis (count $< 1.0 \times 10^9$/L, usually $< 0.2 \times 10^9$/L) should be distinguished from the mild granulocytopenia that can occur in Graves' hyperthyroidism and/or with thionamide therapy.
- Patients with agranulocytosis should be treated with supportive measures such as broad-spectrum antibiotics, according to local protocols, similar to those used for agranulocytosis caused by chemotherapy. Hospitalization can be avoided if close observation outside hospital is possible, unless a high fever develops.
- Thionamides should never be used again in affected patients, as cross-reactivity between drugs approaches 50%.

The use of routine blood counts every 2–4 weeks during thionamide therapy remains controversial. Although blood counts are possibly beneficial, the cost in terms of extra visits and increased anxiety for patients with mild granulocytopenia is high.

Other side effects include rash and urticaria (which can be chronic). Although these are common, they are not forerunners of more serious side effects and may be treated by switching to a different thionamide. Fever, arthralgia, toxic hepatitis and cholestatic jaundice are rare. Mild, transient aminotransferase elevations often occur, particularly with higher doses of propylthiouracil, but it is not clear whether liver function should be monitored during thionamide therapy. Remember, Graves' hyperthyroidism per se may cause urticaria.

In patients taking propylthiouracil on a long-term basis, tests for anti-neutrophil cytoplasmic antibodies (ANCA) are positive in up to 25% of hyperthyroid patients in general and up to 65% of hyperthyroid children. ANCA positivity may sometimes be associated with a clinical vasculitis syndrome, with glomerulonephritis and/or alveolar hemorrhage, and these antibodies should be measured if arthralgias develop.

Radio-iodine (^{131}I) remains the most widely used treatment for hyperthyroidism. β-particles account for 90% of the radiation of ^{131}I, and their extremely short radiation path ensures that only thyroid cells and not the surrounding tissues are damaged. The physical half-life of the drug is 8 days, but because of urinary excretion the biological half-life in the patient is much shorter. Radio-iodine is a suitable treatment for any cause of hyperthyroidism in which there is iodine uptake in the gland, but not for transient (destructive) thyroiditis. Treatment must be administered by specifically licensed practitioners.

Advantages and disadvantages. Radio-iodine is given orally as a drink or capsule and offers definitive painless therapy without the need for hospital admission or surgery. However, the response to treatment is slow (from 1 month to many years) and unpredictable (see Figure 3.2); permanent hypothyroidism occurs in most cases of Graves' disease and in many patients with multinodular goiter. In addition, standard radiation precautions may be difficult in mothers with young children. Radio-iodine that is not taken up by the tissues is excreted in the urine and, in smaller amounts, in saliva and breast milk, so it is not appropriate for nursing mothers.

Dose. ^{131}I doses used in hyperthyroidism are typically in the range of 180–600 MBq (5–16 mCi). Dose calculation based on radio-iodine uptake and estimated thyroid gland size is routine practice in some institutions, but others use fixed dosing as, overall, the outcome appears to differ very little. For radio-iodine or other radionuclide uptake, it is usually necessary to rule out transient (destructive) thyroiditis before treatment. A single dose of ^{131}I is sufficient in 80–90% of patients, although this depends on the dose given (Figure 3.5). Patients who are still hyperthyroid after 6 months may be offered a second dose. Higher doses are often required in large multinodular glands and in patients in whom a rapid response is desirable, such as those with cardiac disease.

Pretreatment with thionamides. Most hyperthyroid patients choosing radio-iodine can be safely treated without prior administration of anti-thyroid drugs. There is good evidence that propylthiouracil given before radio-iodine treatment reduces the efficacy of radio-iodine therapy. A 20% increase in the dose of radio-iodine in previously treated patients, especially those treated with propylthiouracil, therefore seems wise. Propylthiouracil or methimazole/carbimazole should be stopped 4–7 days before radio-iodine therapy. Many clinicians prescribe β-blockers before radio-iodine therapy.

Debilitated patients with severe hyperthyroidism and those with cardiac disease are often pretreated with thionamides before radio-iodine therapy. In such patients, thionamides are often restarted

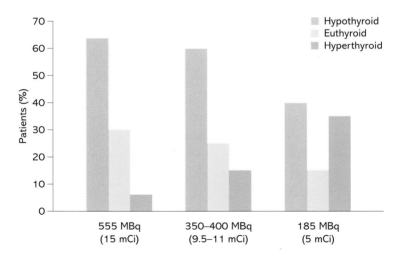

Figure 3.5 Outcomes at 1 year following different doses of radio-iodine. Data from Kendall-Taylor P et al. *BMJ* 1984;289:361–3 and Allahabadia A et al. *J Clin Endocrinol Metab* 2001;86:3611–17.

1 week after radio-iodine therapy while its effects become established. Some clinicians use a 'block–replace' regimen with thyroxine after treatment, as the risk of rapid-onset hypothyroidism is high at this stage. In selected patients with Graves' disease, oral administration of iodine drops (see below) 1 week after radio-iodine treatment accelerates the return to the euthyroid state.

Contraindications to radio-iodine include pregnancy and breastfeeding. Patients are also advised not to become pregnant for 4–12 months (depending on national guidelines) after radio-iodine therapy, and pregnancy testing should be performed routinely before administration. If radio-iodine is inadvertently given in pregnancy, specialist radiation advice should be sought, but it is not necessarily an indication for termination of pregnancy. Radio-iodine should also be used with caution in thyroid eye disease (see page 63). The use of radio-iodine in children remains controversial, but is employed in many centers in the USA. This practice is not widespread in the UK because of concerns over the risk of thyroid cancer (see Side effects below), but it is likely to be safe, at least in older children.

Radiation precautions. To reduce the general radiation exposure to the public, standard precautions are advised (Table 3.6).

Monitoring for hypothyroidism. In some individuals, the onset of hypothyroidism after radio-iodine can occur within 4–6 weeks. Repeat thyroid function testing is advisable at 4 weeks, and then at 2–3-month intervals. T4 levels – not TSH levels (which may remain suppressed for as long as 12 months after treatment of hyperthyroidism, even after the patient has become euthyroid or hypothyroid) – should be used to monitor the response until TSH level becomes detectable. The risk of hypothyroidism continues for up to 20 years, and patients who remain euthyroid after 1 year should continue to have thyroid function tests at 6–12-month intervals, either indefinitely or until thyroxine is required.

If hypothyroidism develops in the first year, full doses of T4 (e.g. 100 µg or 1.6 µg/kg/day) can be used immediately to alleviate symptoms, rather than titrating up from very small doses, as the hypothyroidism is known to be of recent onset. The thyroid is generally no longer palpable when permanent hypothyroidism occurs after radio-iodine therapy for Graves' disease, but transient hypothyroidism

TABLE 3.6

Typical radiation precautions after a 400 MBq dose of radio-iodine

- Do not bring children or anyone who is, or might be, pregnant with you to your appointment

- If you are the main caregiver for young children, you should make arrangements for someone to help care for them if possible; avoid close contact with children for 7 days and limit close contact to no more than 15 minutes daily for the next 2 weeks

- Avoid all close contact with women who are, or may be, pregnant for 7 days, and for the next 2 weeks limit close contact to no more than 15 minutes daily

- Avoid periods of prolonged close contact with other people for 4 days

- Sleep apart from your partner for 4 nights

- For 4 days, avoid staying in places of entertainment or public transportation, where you are likely to be in close contact with other people, for more than 2 hours

- Do not work for 7 days if your work involves close contact with children or women who are or might possibly be pregnant

- Avoid pregnancy or breastfeeding for 4–12 months

Note: precise recommendations may vary between institutions and countries.

(thyroid 'stunning') is common in the first few weeks or months. A persistent goiter or easily palpable thyroid is a clue that 'stunning' rather than permanent hypothyroidism is present.

Side effects. Although external radiation to the neck in children is associated with an increased risk of thyroid nodules and thyroid cancer, large (up to 23 000 patients), long-term (over 26 years) follow-up studies of radio-iodine therapy have shown no major increase in cancer mortality. In one study, overall mortality from cancer was reduced. In some studies, radio-iodine appears to increase the risk of thyroid cancer, but the absolute risk is still very small and appears to be primarily in those treated with radio-iodine for nodular disease rather than for Graves' disease. In the past, patients with hyperthyroidism due to nodular thyroid disease often received radio-iodine without obtaining nodule biopsies, so it is unclear whether the increased cancer risk was the result of radio-iodine therapy or pre-existing malignancies. All suspicious nodules are now biopsied before radio-iodine therapy. Evidence concerning any increase in the incidence of breast, stomach, small-bowel or brain cancer is conflicting; one study has suggested a reduction in lung cancer.

Gonadal exposure after radio-iodine treatment is estimated to be similar to that from a barium enema examination, and there is no evidence of an increased risk of congenital abnormalities in the children of women treated with radio-iodine. Transient exacerbation of thyrotoxicosis, and even thyrotoxic storm, has been reported immediately after treatment with radio-iodine, but the latter is rare. The small (1.2-fold) increased risk of cardiovascular death reported after radio-iodine treatment probably relates to the consequences of hyperthyroidism itself, rather than to radio-iodine therapy.

Other drugs. Thionamides inhibit thyroid hormone synthesis, and are therefore relatively slow in achieving a euthyroid state. Under certain circumstances, additional drugs with different mechanisms of action are used (Table 3.7).

Inhibitors of T4-to-T3 conversion. Drugs that inhibit the peripheral conversion of T4 to T3 are particularly helpful when hyperthyroidism needs to be controlled urgently. Agents originally developed as radio-graphic contrast media, including sodium ipodate and iopanoic acid, are among the most powerful inhibitors of T4-to-T3 conversion (Box 3.1).

Box 3.1

At the time of writing, sodium ipodate is not available in the USA or UK. Iopanoic acid is not available in the USA but, at present, it can be obtained in the UK through a European supplier, and can be used at the same doses as quoted for ipodate. Please note that, despite being very effective, these agents are not indicated for the routine treatment of thyrotoxicosis, and their clinical application, as described in this book, is unlicensed.

TABLE 3.7

Drugs used to treat hyperthyroidism and their mechanism of action

Mechanism of action	Drug
Inhibition of thyroid hormone synthesis	Thionamide drugs
Inhibition of thyroid hormone release	Iodine
	Lithium
Inhibition of T4-to-T3 conversion	Iodinated contrast media (e.g. iopanoic acid)
	Amiodarone*
	Propylthiouracil (weak effect)
	Glucocorticoids (weak effect)
	Propranolol (weak effect)
Inhibition of iodine uptake	Perchlorate
Binding to thyroid hormone in gastrointestinal tract and preventing enterohepatic circulation	Cholestyramine (not routine)
Symptomatic therapy	β-blockers

*Only in conjunction with specialist endocrinologic consultation.

These compounds also release iodine and hence inhibit thyroid hormone release. There is some evidence that they also block the ability of T3 to bind to its receptor.

Overall, a typical dose of 0.5–1.0 g/day produces a rapid reduction of T3 levels, often within 36–72 hours. These inhibitors are seldom used alone (they can be combined with thionamides) or for long-term therapy, because if escape from inhibition occurs, the patient becomes loaded with iodine and the effectiveness of subsequent radio-iodine may be reduced.

However, they are recommended for very rapid control of hyperthyroidism for a short time:

- pending definitive therapy, for example in thyrotoxic storm in combination with thionamides

- in patients with thionamide-induced agranulocytosis before surgery or after radio-iodine therapy
- in severely ill elderly patients with cardiac disease
- in patients with amiodarone-induced thyrotoxicosis awaiting the benefits of amiodarone withdrawal
- as preparation for surgery
- in severely hyperthyroid pregnant women
- in patients with severe destructive thyroiditis or severe hyperthyroidism after T4 overdose.

Propylthiouracil, glucocorticoids and propranolol also inhibit T4-to-T3 conversion, but their effect is too weak to be clinically useful and hence they are not used specifically for this purpose.

Amiodarone is a potent inhibitor of T4-to-T3 conversion, but it must be used only in conjunction with specialist endocrinologic consultation, as it can also induce or exacerbate thyrotoxicosis.

Inhibitors of thyroid hormone release

Inorganic iodide (typically 3 drops of Lugol's solution three times daily [8 mg iodide per drop] or 1–3 drops of supersaturated potassium iodide three times daily [35–50 mg per drop]) improves thyroid function within days by inhibiting the release of thyroid hormones.

Although inorganic iodide does not return the patient to the euthyroid state, it can be effective for prolonged periods in some individuals with relatively mild thyrotoxicosis.

In more severe Graves' disease, the thyroid may escape the inhibitory effect, and in multinodular goiter, the iodine load may exacerbate disease. When thyroid hormone biosynthesis is inhibited with a thionamide, however, iodide is a useful adjunct because of its inhibitory effects on thyroid hormone release.

It is also effective when administered after radio-iodine therapy for Graves' disease, when it can be given as a potassium iodide solution, 3 drops twice daily, 1 week after the administration of radio-iodine.

Inorganic iodide is generally reserved for temporary but rapid reduction in thyroid function pending definitive therapy (e.g. in thyrotoxic storm or preoperative preparation).

Lithium carbonate, 300–450 mg three times daily, inhibits thyroid hormone release and may rapidly control hyperthyroidism in a manner similar to inorganic iodide. Escape from inhibition occurs with prolonged therapy. It can also be used for rapid control of hyperthyroidism in patients who are allergic to iodide, although side effects are common. It has also been advocated as combination therapy with radio-iodine, as it increases thyroidal retention of ^{131}I, but its narrow therapeutic window makes it a less desirable agent.

Inhibitors of iodine uptake

Potassium perchlorate competitively inhibits iodine uptake in the thyroid and reduces thyroid hormone production. As it does not affect the biosynthesis of thyroid hormone, it is given in conjunction with thionamides. Potassium perchlorate is particularly recommended in iodine-induced hyperthyroidism, which is typically a consequence of amiodarone administration, to deplete iodine stores in the thyroid. High doses carry a risk of aplastic anemia and gastric ulceration, but these do not occur very often at conventional doses (1 g/day).

Specific treatment regimens

Thyrotoxic (thyroid) storm. Critically ill hyperthyroid patients should be admitted to hospital. Concomitant illnesses, particularly infection, must be treated. Multidrug therapy directed at different steps in the production and activation of thyroid hormone is detailed below.

- *Inhibition of thyroid hormone biosynthesis.* Propylthiouracil, 200 mg every 4 hours, methimazole, 20 mg every 4 hours or 30 mg every 6 hours, or carbimazole, 25 mg every 4 hours or 40 mg every 6 hours, is administered. Thionamides are not available as parenteral preparations, but may be administered by nasogastric tube or per rectum (propylthiouracil) if necessary.
- *Administration of a β-blocker,* for example propranolol, 40–80 mg every 6 hours, to decrease tachycardia. When hypotension is present, shorter-acting parenteral β-blockers, such as esmolol, may be preferred.
- *Inhibition of T4-to-T3 conversion.* Serum T3 can be normalized with these inhibitors in 36–72 hours. Effects on T4 are less dramatic.

Sodium ipodate (or its equivalent; see Box 3.1, page 58) is typically used in a 2 g loading dose followed by 1 g/day for 1–2 weeks, or longer in certain situations. Amiodarone is the only available parenteral agent that inhibits conversion of T4 to T3 but, as has already been discussed, this must only be used in conjunction with specialist endocrinologic consultation.

- *Inhibition of thyroid hormone release.* Iodine is commonly used, for example as a potassium iodide solution (containing about 35 mg iodide per drop), 3 drops twice daily, or as sodium iodide, 1 g intravenously. The iodine released from iopanoic acid or amiodarone may also serve this purpose.
- *Bile sequestrants* such as cholestyramine may be beneficial by preventing the enterohepatic circulation of thyroid hormone, thereby facilitating its disappearance.
- *Plasmapheresis* may be required in rare circumstances to remove excess thyroid hormone.

Although hydrocortisone, 100 mg every 6 hours, has been suggested as adjunctive therapy, in the absence of concomitant adrenal insufficiency there seems to be little indication for its use.

Once the crisis is over, arrangements for definitive therapy (i.e. radio-iodine or surgery) should be made as soon as possible to prevent a recurrence, particularly in poorly compliant individuals.

Amiodarone-induced thyrotoxicosis. Appropriate therapy is difficult and requires close consultation with an endocrinologist and cardiologist. When the distinction between type 1 (nodular goiter or Graves' disease) and type 2 (destructive thyroiditis) disease is uncertain, glucocorticoids and anti-thyroid drugs are often prescribed together.

Glucocorticoids cause a prompt fall in thyroid hormone concentrations in type 2 disease. Thionamides and perchlorate are useful in type 1 disease. Surgery may be necessary in difficult cases, and preparation is facilitated by adding iopanoic acid to further block conversion of T4 to T3. Radio-iodine is a reasonable choice in the rare type-1 patient with detectable iodine uptake. The advantages and disadvantages of amiodarone discontinuation are still being debated in Type 2 disease.

Thyroid eye disease. Worsening thyroid eye disease can be devastating for patients, so many physicians avoid radio-iodine therapy in patients with moderate or severe active thyroid eye disease (i.e. with moderate-to-severe inflammatory changes, moderate-to-severe proptosis, diplopia or optic nerve compression). Once the disease has reached the 'dry' phase, with low clinical activity scores, some specialists are willing to use radio-iodine. Some clinicians recommend prophylactic glucocorticoid therapy (e.g. prednisone, 30 mg/day for 1 month, 20 mg/day for the second month and 10 mg/day for the third month) for patients with active, mild thyroid eye disease receiving radio-iodine. However, many only prescribe glucocorticoids when eye signs or symptoms worsen.

The overall approach to the treatment of thyroid eye disease is summarized in Table 3.8. Opinions on specific therapy are divided. Some advocate only supportive therapy until the disease is stable for about 1 year, at which time the appearance is corrected surgically with a combination of orbital decompression, strabismus correction and oculoplastic procedures (in that order). Others advocate early immunosuppressive treatment in the active phase of disease to reduce the need for later surgery (Table 3.9). The most commonly used immunosuppressive treatments include glucocorticoids and orbital radiotherapy. Less commonly used immunosuppressants include azathioprine, ciclosporin (cyclosporine), intravenous immunoglobulin and plasmapheresis.

Until more evidence is available, the exact combination of measures will remain controversial, but it is strongly recommended that patients with anything more than mild disease should be assessed and managed jointly by an endocrinologist and an ophthalmologist experienced in this challenging condition. Access to psychological and/or peer support groups is also invaluable (see Useful addresses, page 139), as the distress caused by this disfiguring condition is often underappreciated.

Subclinical hyperthyroidism. Management of patients with endogenous subclinical hyperthyroidism remains controversial in the absence of appropriate intervention trials. Almost all clinicians recommend therapy when there is evidence of associated cardiac disease, atrial fibrillation or

TABLE 3.8

Overall approach to the treatment of thyroid eye disease

Complaint	Treatment for minor symptoms	Treatment for moderate/severe symptoms
Soft tissue swelling and irritation	Avoid salt Dark glasses (preferably wrap-around) Eye lubricants Cold compresses Diuretics Elevate head of bed Tape lids at night	As for minor plus external-beam radiation therapy Glucocorticoids or other immunosuppressants
Proptosis	Cosmetic surgery, e.g. lateral tarsorrhaphy will improve appearance but does not change bulging	Orbital decompression
Extraocular muscles (diplopia)	Prisms in glasses Consider immunosuppression if disease is active	Patch to cover bad eye Immunosuppression and/or external-beam radiotherapy if disease is active Muscle surgery ('burnt-out disease')*
Corneal involvement	Tape lids at night	Orbital decompression
Loss of vision due to optic nerve involvement		Orbital decompression External radiation Glucocorticoids or other immunosuppressants

*When proptosis is severe, concomitant orbital decompression may be necessary.

osteoporosis. Patients with nodular disease are commonly treated with radio-iodine, as are most elderly patients with Graves' disease with TSH levels below 0.1 mU/L; many clinicians recommend therapy for such elderly patients even when they are asymptomatic. Observation is

TABLE 3.9

An approach to treatment of thyroid eye disease favoring immunosuppression

Disease stage	Active 'wet' disease	'Burnt-out, dry' disease
Mild – 'grittiness', irritation, mild proptosis	Lubricants, topical glucocorticoids or non-steroidal agents	Oculoplastic procedures to improve appearance if required
Moderate – as mild but with moderate proptosis and periorbital/ conjunctival edema	Consider low-dose glucocorticoids, e.g. prednisolone, 10–15 mg for 1–2 months	As mild
Marked – as moderate but with marked proptosis, restricted eye movements and diplopia	Combination immunosuppression, e.g. orbital radiotherapy, prednisolone, 30 mg, azathioprine or ciclosporin	Orbital decompression and/or strabismus surgery
Severe – signs of optic nerve compression	Immediate intravenous methylprednisolone, 500 mg/day for 2–3 doses, then as for marked disease*	Urgent orbital decompression

*Lower doses (e.g. 100 mg daily by mouth) are more commonly employed in the USA. Table provided courtesy of MJ Potts.

a reasonable course of action in younger asymptomatic patients, but many clinicians recommend treatment if the hyperthyroidism persists for 6–12 months. Anti-thyroid drugs may also be used, but will not work in the long term for nodular disease.

Although the consequences of mildly subnormal serum TSH are unknown, therapy is sometimes recommended for patients with serum TSH levels of 0.1–0.2 mU/L, particularly elderly patients with nodular disease and those with cardiac disease or osteoporosis.

Surgical management

Thyroidectomy is the oldest form of treatment for hyperthyroidism. Most thyroid surgeons now perform near-total thyroidectomy, leaving behind 5 g or less of thyroid tissue, which reduces the risk of recurrence of hyperthyroidism, but makes hypothyroidism almost inevitable. In inexperienced hands it also increases the risk of the two main complications: recurrent laryngeal nerve palsy and permanent hypocalcemia.

In experienced centers, the incidence of these complications and of postoperative hemorrhage should be less than 1%, and it is

---

Key points – hyperthyroidism: diagnosis and management

- Confirmation of hyperthyroidism is based on measurement of TSH, T4, free T4 and T3, while radionuclide scanning is helpful for differential diagnosis.
- Thyrotoxicosis that develops within 9 months of parturition may be due to postpartum thyroiditis and may be self-limiting (see Chapter 6).
- Medical therapy with thionamides normalizes thyroid function in 4–6 weeks and may induce remission in Graves' hyperthyroidism after 12–18 months in 50–60% of cases; if relapse occurs, the definitive therapy is radio-iodine or surgery.
- Both radio-iodine and thyroidectomy for Graves' hyperthyroidism usually lead to hypothyroidism. In inexperienced hands, thyroidectomy carries a high risk of recurrent laryngeal nerve palsy and permanent hypocalcemia.
- Although subclinical hyperthyroidism is more common than hyperthyroidism itself, management remains controversial in the absence of appropriate intervention trials.
- Management of thyroid eye disease remains challenging, and patients should be managed jointly by an endocrinologist and an ophthalmologist with experience in this condition; the disfigurement and psychological distress it causes is often underestimated.

recommended that thyroidectomy is only performed by surgeons with extensive experience of the technique. Keloid scar formation is an additional concern in susceptible patients.

Appropriate preoperative preparation is essential for hyperthyroid patients. This traditionally includes thionamide treatment until the patient is near-euthyroid (i.e. T4 and/or T3 levels within the reference range irrespective of TSH). Potassium iodide solution, 3–20 drops/day, is given 10 days before surgery for Graves' disease to decrease the vascularity of the thyroid gland.

An alternative approach is to use β-blockade alone in sufficiently high doses to maintain the pulse at less than 90 beats/minute; this may require up to 1 g/day of propranolol. When thionamides are not used, iopanoic acid may be added to β-blockers 3–5 days before surgery.

The current indications for thyroidectomy are shown in Table 3.10, but may depend upon the availability of an experienced surgeon. Some surgeons recommend thyroidectomy under local anesthesia, as a day case in some situations, but this requires additional evaluation.

TABLE 3.10

Indications for thyroidectomy in hyperthyroidism

- Patient preference, e.g. fear of radio-iodine
- Children (radio-iodine and prolonged drug treatment are also viable options)
- Pregnancy (treatment with thionamides is usually preferred)
- Large goiter (particularly multinodular goiter, with local compressive symptoms)
- Severe reaction to anti-thyroid drugs (radio-iodine is also an option)
- Severe ophthalmopathy (thionamides are also an option)
- Suspicious nodule (diagnosed by fine-needle aspiration cytology) plus hyperthyroidism
- Complex situations in which other treatments have failed, e.g. poor compliance with anti-thyroid drugs when radio-iodine is refused

Key references

AACE Thyroid Task Force. American Association of Clinical Endocrinologists. Medical guidelines for clinical practice for the evaluation and treatment of hyperthyroidism and hypothyroidism. *Endocr Pract* 2002;8:457–69.

Abraham P, Avenell A, Watson WA et al. Antithyroid drug regimen for treating Graves' hyperthyroidism. *Cochrane Database Syst Rev* 2004;2:CD003420. The Cochrane Library, issue 1. Chichester: John Wiley & Sons, 2005 (www.thecochranelibrary.com)

Arbelle JE, Porath A. Practice guidelines for the detection and management of thyroid dysfunction. A comparative review of the recommendations. *Clin Endocrinol (Oxf)* 1999;51:11–18.

Bartalena L, Marcocci C, Bogazzi F et al. Relation between therapy for hyperthyroidism and the course of Graves' ophthalmopathy. *N Engl J Med* 1998;338:73–8.

Cooper DS. Hyperthyroidism. *Lancet* 2003;362:459–68.

Cooper DS, Antithyroid drugs. *N Engl J Med* 2005;3:905–17.

Fontanilla JC, Scheider AB, Sarne DH. The use of oral radiographic contrast agents in the management of hyperthyroidism. *Thyroid* 2001;11:561–7.

Franklyn JA, Maisonneuve P, Sheppard M et al. Cancer incidence and mortality after radio-iodine treatment for hyperthyroidism: a population-based cohort study. *Lancet* 1999;353:2111–15.

Leech NJ, Dayan CM. Controversies in the management of Graves' disease. *Clin Endocrinol (Oxf)* 1998;49:273–80.

Maugendre D, Gatel A, Campion L et al. Antithyroid drugs and Graves' disease – prospective randomized assessment of long-term treatment. *Clin Endocrinol (Oxf)* 1999;50: 127–32.

Mourits MP, Prummel MF, Wiersinga WM et al. Clinical activity score as a guide in the management of patients with Graves' ophthalmopathy. *Clin Endocrinol (Oxf)* 1997;47:9–14.

Osman F, Gammage MD, Sheppard MC, Franklyn JA. Cardiac dysrhythmias and thyroid dysfunction: the hidden menace? *J Clin Endocrinol Metab* 2002; 87:963–7.

Surks MI, Ortiz E, Daniels GH et al. Subclinical thyroid disease: scientific review and guidelines for diagnosis and management. *JAMA* 2004; 291:228–38.

Torring O, Tallstedt L, Wallin G et al. Graves' hyperthyroidism: treatment with antithyroid drugs, surgery, or radio-iodine – a prospective randomized study. Thyroid Study Group. *J Clin Endocrinol Metab* 1996;81:2986–93.

Hypothyroidism: etiology and presentation

Hypothyroidism is a syndrome of thyroid hormone deficiency and its clinical consequences. Primary hypothyroidism, which results from damage to, inhibition of, or removal of the thyroid itself, is very common. Secondary forms of hypothyroidism (central hypothyroidism), arising from hypothalamic or pituitary disorders, are rare.

This chapter looks at the etiology and clinical features of overt primary hypothyroidism, mild (subclinical) hypothyroidism and secondary hypothyroidism. The diagnosis and management of these conditions are discussed in Chapter 5.

Etiology of primary hypothyroidism

Iodine deficiency as a cause of hypothyroidism is rare in the USA and uncommon in Western Europe. However, between the early 1970s and early 1990s the median iodine intake in the USA decreased by 50%, with 15% of women of childbearing age having borderline iodide deficiency.

Iatrogenic hypothyroidism results from surgical thyroidectomy, radio-iodine therapy for hyperthyroidism and external-beam radiation therapy for head and neck malignancies. Potentially reversible hypothyroidism may occur after long-term administration of medications such as lithium and those containing iodine, for example amiodarone. Transient or potentially reversible hypothyroidism also occurs in many forms of destructive thyroiditis (such as postviral subacute thyroiditis and postpartum thyroiditis), as a consequence of thyroid 'stunning' soon after radio-iodine therapy for Graves' disease and after subtotal thyroid resection.

Chronic autoimmune thyroiditis is the most common cause of spontaneous primary hypothyroidism in iodine-sufficient regions.

The condition is known as Hashimoto's thyroiditis if goiter is present and atrophic thyroiditis if the size of the thyroid is diminished.

Hashimoto's thyroiditis

Hashimoto's thyroiditis, also known as autoimmune thyroiditis and chronic lymphocytic thyroiditis, is a genetic autoimmune disorder most commonly seen in women. Postpartum thyroiditis is a variant of Hashimoto's thyroiditis (see Chapter 6).

The prevalence of Hashimoto's thyroiditis correlates with iodine intake, with higher prevalences in areas of high iodine intake. Animal models show that dietary iodine is required for the expression of auto-immune thyroiditis, whereas low dietary iodine prevents thyroiditis. In humans with Hashimoto's thyroiditis, exposure to high concentrations of iodine (e.g. from amiodarone, iodinated contrast material or potassium iodide) may inhibit thyroid hormone synthesis and release, worsening hypothyroidism. Lithium also inhibits the release of thyroid hormone, with almost one-third of patients treated with this agent developing transient hypothyroidism. However, severe or permanent lithium-induced hypothyroidism suggests underlying autoimmune thyroiditis.

Autoimmune thyroid disease, including Hashimoto's thyroiditis, can be precipitated by several immunotherapeutic agents, particularly in patients with anti-thyroid antibodies.

These agents include:
- recombinant human interferon α (particularly when treating hepatitis C)
- recombinant human interferon β
- interleukin-2
- granuloctye colony-stimulating factor (G-CSF) (possibly).

Subclinical hypothyroidism

Widespread laboratory testing for thyroid dysfunction has shown that most hypothyroid patients have mild (subclinical) hypothyroidism. In the Whickham study, a long-term prospective study of thyroid function, subclinical hypothyroidism was found in 8% of women and 3% of men. Its prevalence increases with age: 10–20% of women and

5–10% of men over 65 years old have an elevated serum thyroid-stimulating hormone (TSH) (the majority below 10 mU/L). Many, but not all, patients with subclinical hypothyroidism progress to overt hypothyroidism.

- Women with an elevated serum TSH and positive anti-thyroid antibodies develop overt hypothyroidism at a rate of 4.3% per year.
- Women with elevated TSH alone develop the condition at a rate of 2.6% per year.
- Women with positive antibodies only, develop overt hypothyroidism at a rate of 2.1% per year.

Conversely, serum TSH returns to normal over 4 years in 20–30% of patients with serum TSH levels of 5–10 mU/L.

Etiology. Most patients with subclinical hypothyroidism have anti-thyroid antibodies, confirming the diagnosis of Hashimoto's thyroiditis. In a small group of patients of varying ages, subclinical hypothyroidism is caused by inactivating mutations in the TSH receptor, or defects of biosynthesis of thyroid hormone (e.g. Pendred's syndrome).

Secondary hypothyroidism

Hypothyroidism due to hypothalamic or pituitary disease is known as secondary or central hypothyroidism. These secondary forms of hypothyroidism are rare; hypopituitarism, of which secondary hypothyroidism is a component, occurs in only one in every 10 000 individuals.

Etiology. Diseases that affect the pituitary and hypothalamus often involve multiple pituitary hormones, including gonadotropins, adrenocorticotropic hormone (ACTH) and TSH. Secondary hypothyroidism can result from surgery on, or external-beam radiation to, the pituitary (or hypothalamus), or from inflammatory disorders involving the hypothalamus and pituitary. Transient central hypothyroidism may result during bexarotene therapy for cutaneous T-cell lymphoma.

Clinical presentation of hypothyroidism

Non-specific symptoms. The severity of clinical signs and symptoms in hypothyroid patients is generally proportional to the degree of thyroid hormone deficiency and its duration. Many of the symptoms are non-specific (Table 4.1).

TABLE 4.1

Signs and symptoms of hypothyroidism

Symptoms	Signs
General	
Modest weight gain	Hypothermia*
Cold intolerance	
Decreased energy	
Cutaneous	
Cold, dry, puffy skin	Cold, dry, puffy skin
Hair loss	Periorbital puffiness
	Myxedema* (non-pitting edema)
	Carotinemia*
	Hair loss (scalp and lateral eyebrows)
	Vitiligo[†]
	Alopecia areata[†]
Head, ears, eyes, nose, throat	
Proptosis[‡]	Enlarged tongue*
Hoarseness*	
Decreased hearing[†]	
Respiratory	
Exertional dyspnea	Pleural effusions*
	Sleep apnea*
Cardiovascular	
	Bradycardia*
	Diastolic hypertension*
	Pericardial effusion*
	Congestive heart failure**

TABLE 4.1 (CONTINUED)

Signs and symptoms of hypothyroidism

Symptoms	Signs
Thyroid gland	
Sense of neck pressure from goiter	Enlarged[†] Atrophic
Gastrointestinal	
Constipation	Ascites* Ileus*
Neuromuscular	
Muscle pain, stiffness, cramps Paresthesias Impaired cognition Dementia* Coma*,**	Delayed relaxation of deep tendon reflexes Enlarged muscles* Cerebellar ataxia*
Skeletal	
Carpal tunnel syndrome* Joint discomfort, arthralgias	Joint effusions*
Genitourinary	
Metrorrhagia Amenorrhea Infertility Galactorrhea* Erectile dysfunction	Breast discharge*
Psychiatric	
Depression Apathy Psychosis*,**	

*Generally found only with severe hypothyroidism.
[†]Found in patients with an autoimmune condition that may be associated with Hashimoto's thyroiditis.
[‡]May occur with Hashimoto's thyroiditis, but much more common with Graves' disease.
**Extremely rare.

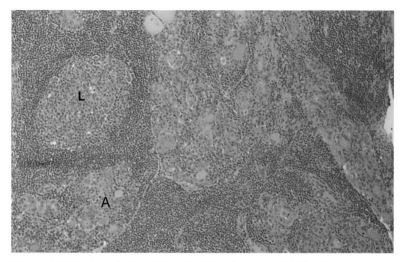

Figure 4.1 Hashimoto's thyroiditis with diffuse lymphocytic infiltration. L, lymphoid follicle; A, follicular epithelium with oxyphil change. Printed courtesy of Dr Wanda Szyfelbein.

Both euthyroid and mildly hypothyroid individuals may complain of fatigue, weight gain, dry skin, mental torpor, depression or constipation. Muscle cramps, joint pains, menorrhagia or infertility may be unrecognized clues to the presence of hypothyroidism. Marked obesity, or relentless weight gain, is seldom caused by hypothyroidism. The clinical diagnosis of hypothyroidism is often unreliable. Symptoms can only be attributed to hypothyroidism when accompanied by laboratory confirmation of thyroid hormone deficiency (see Chapter 5).

Hashimoto's thyroiditis. The thyroid gland is diffusely infiltrated with lymphocytes, and the thyroid follicular cells develop an oxyphilic appearance, so-called Hurthle cells (Figure 4.1). The thyroid gland is generally enlarged, non-tender and firmer than normal, with a bosselated or pebbly surface. It is easy for the clinician to misinterpret the firm lobe of Hashimoto's thyroiditis as a nodule, but discrete thyroid nodules must be evaluated even when Hashimoto's thyroiditis is present. The thyroid ranges in size from normal to much larger than normal.

Autoantibodies with an affinity for thyroid-specific antigens are the laboratory hallmark of Hashimoto's thyroiditis. Anti-thyroid peroxidase antibodies and/or antithyroglobulin antibodies are found in almost all patients, and are a good diagnostic indicator for this condition. Antibodies that interact with and possibly block the TSH receptor, and antibodies against the sodium iodide symporter, may also be present. Antibodies against T4 and T3 can interfere with their measurement.

The natural history of Hashimoto's thyroiditis is quite variable. Some patients slowly develop progressive hypothyroidism, but a smaller number with moderate or even severe hypothyroidism eventually become euthyroid. Hypothyroid patients may recover after the loss of TSH-receptor-blocking antibodies, removal of a causative agent (such as iodine) or recovery from various forms of destructive thyroiditis.

Proptosis (exophthalmos) and other manifestations of thyroid eye disease can occur in patients with Hashimoto's thyroiditis, but they are generally less severe than in patients with Graves' disease. Hyperglobulinemia, positive antinuclear antibodies, elevated erythrocyte sedimentation rate and monoclonal antibody patterns may accompany otherwise uncomplicated Hashimoto's thyroiditis.

Associated conditions. A number of other autoimmune disorders are associated with Hashimoto's thyroiditis (Table 4.2), including vitamin B_{12} deficiency. It is therefore reasonable to measure serum

TABLE 4.2

Common and uncommon autoimmune disorders associated with Hashimoto's thyroiditis

Common	Uncommon
• Premature gray hair	• Addison's disease
• Vitiligo	• Type 1 diabetes mellitus
• Vitamin B_{12} deficiency	• Celiac disease
	• Dermatitis herpetiformis
	• Multiple sclerosis
	• Rheumatoid arthritis
	• Systemic lupus erythematosus
	• Systemic sclerosis

B_{12} concentration periodically in patients with autoimmune thyroid disease, because B_{12} deficiency is easy to treat.

Recent literature has popularized a central nervous system disorder called Hashimoto's encephalopathy. This disorder responds to glucocorticoids, has associated anti-thyroid antibodies and may be an autoimmune disease; however, Hashimoto's thyroiditis does not *cause* this malady.

Complications

Myxedema crisis is a rare phenomenon in which patients with profound hypothyroidism (myxedema) may become critically ill, often after unrelated hospital admissions. The various metabolic effects of myxedema, including impaired free-water excretion, decreased carbon dioxide-stimulated respiratory drive and impaired drug metabolism, contribute to clinical deterioration or coma (Table 4.3). Already somnolent patients with myxedema may deteriorate further when exposed to sedatives, tranquilizers or narcotics. Profound hypothyroidism also impairs the pituitary gland's ACTH response to stress, resulting in relative or absolute cortisol deficiency and acute adrenal insufficiency.

TABLE 4.3

Metabolic disturbances of myxedema crisis

- Hypoventilation
- Hyponatremia
- Hypothermia
- Hypometabolism of drugs
- Hyporesponse to infection (no febrile response)
- Hypoglycemia
- Hypoadrenocorticism
- Hypotension
- Hypotonia of the bowel (constipation)
- Hypothyroidism

Subclinical hypothyroidism. In some clinical studies, patients with subclinical hypothyroidism experience more hypothyroid symptoms than euthyroid individuals, but fewer than those with overt hypothyroidism. However, not all patients have symptoms.

Central hypothyroidism. The possibility of central hypothyroidism should be considered in patients who present with symptoms characteristic of hypothyroidism in association with hypogonadism (amenorrhea) or signs of adrenal insufficiency.

Key points – hypothyroidism: etiology and presentation

- The severity of hypothyroid clinical signs and symptoms is generally proportional to the degree of thyroid hormone deficiency and its duration; many of the symptoms are non-specific.
- In iodine-sufficient regions, chronic autoimmune thyroiditis (known as Hashimoto's disease if goiter is present or atrophic thyroiditis if thyroid size is diminished) is the most common cause of spontaneous primary hypothyroidism.
- Subclinical hypothyroidism is very common, particularly among the elderly.
- Secondary hypothyroidism is usually due to structural hypothalamic or pituitary disease, and may be associated with deficiency of other hormones, including gonadotropins and adrenocorticotropic hormone.

Key references

Cooper DS. Clinical practice. Subclinical hypothyroidism. *N Engl J Med* 2001;345:260–5.

Dayan CM, Daniels GH. Chronic autoimmune thyroiditis. *N Engl J Med* 1996;335:99–107.

Hollowell JG, Staehling NW, Hannon WH et al. Iodine nutrition in the United States. Trends and public health implications: iodine excretion data from National Health and Nutrition Examination Surveys I and III (1971–1974 and 1988–1994). *J Clin Endocrinol Metab* 1998;83: 3401–8.

Jenkins RC, Weetman AP. Disease associations with autoimmune thyroid disease. *Thyroid* 2002; 12:977–88.

Laurberg P, Nohr SB, Pedersen KM et al. Thyroid disorders in mild iodine deficiency. *Thyroid* 2000;10: 951–63.

Lindsay RS, Toft AD. Hypothyroidism. *Lancet* 1997; 349:413–17.

Vanderpump MPJ, Tunbridge WMG, French JM et al. The incidence of thyroid disorders in the community: a twenty-year follow-up of the Whickham Survey. *Clin Endocrinol (Oxf)* 1995;43:55–68.

Diagnosis

Biochemical confirmation of primary hypothyroidism. The earliest and most sensitive sign of a failing thyroid gland is a rising level of thyroid-stimulating hormone (TSH), as TSH elevation occurs well before serum T4, free T4 or T3 levels fall below the normal range (Figure 5.1). Measurement of serum TSH, usually in conjunction with serum free T4, should be the mainstay of thyroid testing strategies. Serum T3 is not a reliable indicator of hypothyroidism, as it may remain normal a long way into the development of the condition; conversely, low T3 levels often occur in non-thyroidal illness.

Many biochemical abnormalities, resulting from a wide range of metabolic disturbances, occur in patients with profound hypothyroidism, and may provide important diagnostic clues.

- Elevated blood levels of creatine phosphokinase, liver amino-transferases, amylase, myoglobin, homocysteine, and total and low-density lipoprotein (LDL) cholesterol are reversible manifestations of severe hypothyroidism.
- Serum sodium concentration may decline, with adverse clinical consequences.
- Anemia can be microcytic and hypochromic (secondary to iron deficiency from menorrhagia), macrocytic (in some cases secondary to concomitant vitamin B_{12} deficiency) or normocytic.
- Common electrocardiographic abnormalities include decreased voltage of the QRS complex, and non-specific ST- and T-wave abnormalities.

Concentrations of the cardiac isozyme of creatine phosphokinase and troponin are generally normal in hypothyroidism, ruling out a spurious diagnosis of myocardial infarction. However, long-standing, profound hypothyroidism does predispose patients to coronary artery disease because of its effects on blood pressure, lipid profiles and homocysteine. Compensatory hypertrophy of the pituitary gland (TSH-

79

secreting cells) may appear to mimic a pituitary tumor on magnetic resonance imaging (MRI); the elevated serum prolactin that can accompany severe hypothyroidism may compound this confusion.

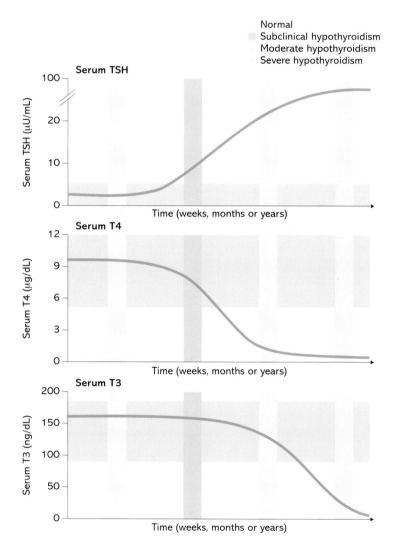

Figure 5.1 Changes in thyroid function during development of primary hypothyroidism. Modified from Ridgway EC. In: *Clinical Thyroid Disease Management*. Deerfield, Illinois: Flint Laboratories, 1987.

Hashimoto's thyroiditis. A firm, symmetrically enlarged thyroid gland, in association with anti-thyroid antibodies and a high normal or elevated serum TSH level is virtually diagnostic of Hashimoto's thyroiditis. If a thyroid nodule is suspected, thyroid ultrasonography may be used to resolve the uncertainty. On ultrasound scans, the thyroid in Hashimoto's thyroiditis appears heterogeneous and hypoechoic, and may be misinterpreted as a thyroid with multiple small nodules. When a discrete nodule is found, a fine-needle aspirate biopsy should be obtained, even if positive thyroid autoantibodies are present. Radionuclide scans are generally unnecessary, and can be more confusing than helpful, as 24-hour radio-iodine uptake may be low, normal or elevated, with a homogeneous or extremely heterogeneous pattern of tracer uptake.

Diagnosis of Hashimoto's thyroiditis may be important even if thyroid function is normal, as the presence of anti-thyroid antibodies, even with a normal serum TSH level, predicts an increased risk of miscarriage, postpartum thyroiditis (see Chapter 6) and progression to overt hypothyroidism. When Hashimoto's thyroiditis has been diagnosed, aggressive case-finding for autoimmune thyroid disease among the patient's first-degree relatives should be encouraged.

Although lymphoma of the thyroid is rare, it is 80 times more common in patients with Hashimoto's thyroiditis than in the general population. Sudden enlargement of the Hashimoto's thyroid suggests this diagnosis.

Subclinical hypothyroidism. The biochemical features of mild or subclinical hypothyroidism are:
- elevated serum TSH (the earliest sign of a failing thyroid)
- normal concentrations of T4 and free T4
- normal T3 and free T3 (though they not usually measured).

Subclinical hypothyroidism must be distinguished from other causes of a mildly elevated serum TSH. These include:
- untreated primary adrenal insufficiency (Addison's disease)
- the recovery phase of the 'euthyroid-sick' syndrome
- heterophilic antibodies, for example against mouse proteins, which give falsely high TSH values in some assays
- laboratory or clerical error.

Paradoxically, some patients with central hypothyroidism (see below) have a mildly elevated serum TSH as a result of decreased bioactivity; this elevated serum TSH level occurs only when serum free T4 concentrations are very low.

A significant rise in LDL cholesterol occurs as hypothyroidism progresses, particularly when serum TSH exceeds 10 mU/L.

Secondary hypothyroidism. Differentiating primary and secondary (central) hypothyroidism is usually straightforward. Patients with primary hypothyroidism have an elevated serum TSH concentration, while those with pituitary disease have a low serum TSH concentration. However, some moderately to severely hypothyroid patients with hypothalamic–pituitary disease have mildly elevated serum TSH concentrations.

Under normal physiological circumstances, thyroid-releasing hormone (TRH) stimulates not only the release of TSH but also its appropriate glycosylation, which is necessary for TSH to be biologically active. When free T4 concentrations are very low, TSH may be secreted even in the absence of TRH, but is biologically inactive. When the hypothalamic–pituitary–thyroid physiology is intact, an inverse logarithmic relationship exists between free T4 and TSH.

With pituitary or hypothalamic disease, this relationship is broken. Whereas in mild primary hypothyroidism, marked TSH elevation accompanies low free T4 concentrations, in hypothalamic disease TSH is mildly elevated only when free T4 concentrations are very low. A low free T4 and slight TSH elevation may also occur transiently after therapy for hyperthyroidism, as pituitary TSH secretion recovers.

Central hypothyroidism is generally a consequence of structural disease involving the hypothalamus or pituitary gland. Once central hypothyroidism has been diagnosed, it is important to obtain radiological images of this region – usually by MRI – and to evaluate the adequacy of other pituitary hormones.

Evaluation of the hypothalamic–pituitary–adrenal axis is particularly important.

Medical management of primary hypothyroidism

Overall aims. The goals of thyroid hormone therapy for primary hypothyroidism include:

- normalization of serum TSH
- alleviation of symptoms
- prevention of overtreatment.

Normalization of serum TSH is easy to achieve in compliant patients, but specific or non-specific symptoms may persist despite a normal serum TSH concentration. Nevertheless, serum TSH measurement is still the most important guide to appropriate therapy, with the goal being a serum TSH level in the lower half of the normal range (0.45–5.0 mU/L).

Persistent overtreatment, characterized by serum TSH below 0.1 mU/L, may cause adverse consequences, including thinning of the bones (particularly in estrogen-deficient women) and an increased risk of atrial arrhythmias (particularly in the elderly). It is uncertain whether minimally subnormal serum TSH concentrations are of any clinical consequence. Free T4 and TSH should be measured in patients whose TSH concentrations fluctuate without apparent explanation. Poorly compliant patients who have recently restarted their thyroid hormone often have normal free T4 concentrations with high TSH, as TSH takes some time to reach its nadir.

T4 therapy is not recommended for euthyroid individuals who complain of symptoms suggestive of hypothyroidism; a recent study showed no benefit in such individuals. Unless toxic doses are utilized, T4 therapy does not produce weight loss. Preliminary studies suggest that T4 suppressive therapy may be beneficial for euthyroid patients with refractory urticaria who have anti-thyroid antibodies.

Choice of thyroid hormone therapy. T4 is the drug of choice for thyroid hormone therapy because of its:

- ease of administration
- relatively low cost
- therapeutic efficacy.

As T4 is available in many proprietary and generic preparations, a reassessment of thyroid function after switching from one preparation or brand to another is recommended. The long half-life of T4 (7 days) means that once-daily administration is sufficient, and missed doses can be made up by adding to subsequent doses. Patients who are poorly compliant can be given seven doses once weekly by a visiting nurse. Hospitalized patients who are unable to take medications by mouth for more than 1–2 days should receive 75–80% of the oral dose intravenously. In countries in which intravenous T4 is difficult to obtain, such as the UK, it may be safer to administer T4 via a nasogastric tube rather than use the more readily available intravenous T3 preparation.

Some professional and lay individuals argue that appropriate thyroid hormone replacement therapy should include supplemental T3 as well as T4. This view is supported by the results of a short-term trial in which patients receiving T4 plus T3 felt better (using a variety of psychometric indices) than those using T4 alone, although there were no significant improvements in cognitive function. These findings were not confirmed, however, in several other trials in patients with lower initial T4 concentrations. Many questions concerning the longer-term efficacy, safety and optimum regimen of a T4/T3 combination remain unanswered.

Dosage requirement. The full replacement dose of T4 in an athyreotic patient is approximately 1.6 µg/kg/day (mean 112 µg/day; median 125 µg/day) (Table 5.1). The dose of T4 required to normalize serum TSH is proportional to the baseline TSH elevation, and lower doses will often suffice in patients with mild hypothyroidism. In young hypothyroid patients without known or suspected cardiac disease, full replacement doses of T4 can be prescribed. In the elderly and in those with known or suspected cardiac disease, more cautious administration of T4 is recommended, often starting with doses of 12.5–25 µg/day. Lifelong T4 therapy is generally required for patients with moderate or severe hypothyroidism. Even when transient hypothyroidism is suspected, treatment is usually appropriate for symptomatic patients, even if only for a limited time.

It is preferable to ingest T4 on an empty stomach and to avoid coadministration of various vitamins and supplements (particularly those containing iron, calcium or aluminum), which may interfere with

TABLE 5.1

General guidance for T4 therapy in primary hypothyroidism

- Full replacement dose for an athyreotic individual is 1.6 µg/kg/day
- T4 requirement is proportional to basal TSH elevation
- Start younger patients with full replacement dose
- Start therapy in the elderly and in those with pre-existing or suspected cardiac disease at a lower dose (e.g. 12.5–25 µg/day)
- T4 should preferably be taken on an empty stomach
- Vitamins and supplements should not be taken at the same time as T4
- Use serum TSH concentration to monitor therapy

absorption of T4 (Table 5.2). At least 1 hour should separate ingestion of these agents and T4. Inhibition of T4 absorption by food is modest and is in part dependent on the type of food.

T4 clearance is increased by phenytoin, carbamazepine, rifampicin and phenobarbital (see Table 5.2), resulting in up to a 100% rise in T4 requirement. In patients with borderline hypothyroidism, these drugs may precipitate overt hypothyroidism.

The requirement for T4 goes up during pregnancy by as much as 50%, and generally by at least 35 µg/day; the increased requirement is greater in those without any endogenous thyroid function. Other factors that increase the requirement for T4 are shown in Table 5.2.

When no apparent mechanism can be found to explain an increasing T4 requirement, or markedly variable serum TSH concentrations are measured, poor adherence/compliance must be suspected. Adequacy of absorption may be confirmed by first administering 1 mg of levothyroxine by mouth and then measuring the rise in free T4 concentration over the subsequent hours.

Androgen therapy in women decreases the requirement for T4, although the mechanism is uncertain.

The requirement for T4 also seems to decline in the elderly, but this effect is less striking when the decrease in bodyweight with age is considered.

TABLE 5.2

Factors that increase T4 requirement in patients with primary hypothyroidism

Factor	Cause
Pregnancy	TBG excess; possibly other mechanisms as well
Increased metabolism	Phenytoin Carbamazepine Rifampicin Phenobarbital
Decreased absorption	Drug binding* – cholestyramine – iron products – aluminum hydroxide – calcium carbonate – sucralfate – kayexelate[†] – raloxifene Food in general (possibly soy products and fiber) Gastrointestinal disorders – sprue (celiac disease) – miscellaneous gut disorders resulting in malabsorption – short bowel, including jejuno-ilial bypass – absent gut flora (neomycin enteritis)* – jejunal feeding
Increased loss	Protein loss[‡] – nephrotic syndrome
Uncertain mechanism	Estrogens (possibly TBG excess) Sertraline hydrochloride[†] Lovastatin[†]
Worsening hypothyroidism	Spontaneous Drugs that inhibit thyroid function (iodides, lithium, amiodarone) Smoking

*Zinc and selenium salts have not been studied but would be expected to inhibit absorption.
[†]Limited data.
[‡]Chronic gastrointestinal bleeding has not been studied but would be expected to cause loss of thyroid hormone.

Monitoring therapy. It takes approximately five half-lives for a drug to equilibrate, so serum TSH should be measured at least 5 weeks after the last change in T4 dosage. Once stabilized, serum TSH can be measured yearly. It is important to recognize how TSH measurements exaggerate changes in thyroid status. If serum TSH rises from 2 mU/L to 10 mU/L, modest increments of T4 (e.g. 12.5–25 µg/day) are likely to normalize serum TSH. Similarly, if TSH falls from 2.0 mU/L to 0.15 mU/L, a 12.5–25 µg decrease in T4 dosage is likely to normalize serum TSH. A useful algorithm for monitoring T4 treatment is given in Figure 5.2.

- For most asymptomatic hypothyroid patients, TSH only needs to be measured yearly.
- For most hypothyroid patients on replacement levothyroxine serum, measurement of TSH alone is sufficient to guide therapy.
- For poorly compliant patients, measurement of serum TSH and free T4 together is helpful.

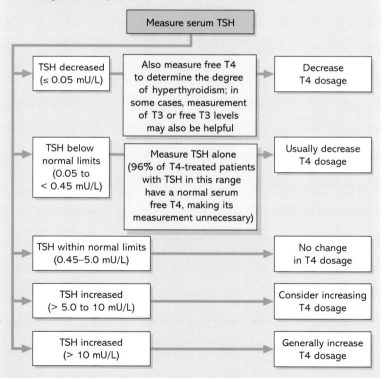

Figure 5.2 An algorithm for monitoring T4 treatment of primary hypothyroidism.

A rise in TSH level in a T4-treated patient may occur as the underlying disease that is causing hypothyroidism progresses, or after the administration of drugs containing iodine or lithium. When the total T4 requirement exceeds 1.6–1.8 µg/kg/day, however, problems with absorption or compliance must be considered.

Optimizing therapy. Although thyroid function can be precisely monitored, not all 'optimally treated' patients feel well. For example, in one study in which patients were treated with increments of thyroid hormone, those whose T4 dose was increased by 25–50 µg/day, resulting in a suppressed serum TSH, felt consistently better than those receiving the highest dose at which TSH could be maintained within the normal range. In another community population-based study, patients taking T4 felt psychologically less well than a matched control population. Several explanations are possible.

- Some of these patients may have been subtly undertreated. When hypothyroid patients remain symptomatic, the T4 dose should be increased until TSH reaches the lower normal range.
- The patients may have remained symptomatic because their symptoms were related to other disorders possibly associated with Hashimoto's thyroiditis, such as depression.
- True physiological replacement of thyroid hormone may require both T4 and T3.
- There could have been ascertainment bias within the study – that is, preferential testing for thyroid disorders in those patients with more complaints.

Clinical deterioration after starting T4 therapy should raise the question of concomitant adrenal insufficiency, known as Schmidt's syndrome.

Treatment of myxedema crisis

Myxedema crisis has been treated with many different therapeutic regimens. Slow replacement therapy is recommended for elderly, profoundly hypothyroid patients who are not critically ill. Profoundly hypothyroid patients who are critically ill require special attention.

Hyponatremia, cortisol deficiency, carbon dioxide retention, use of sedating drugs, hypoglycemia and infection must be recognized and treated aggressively in an intensive therapy unit.

Specific regimens. As severe illness impairs the peripheral conversion of T4 to T3, regimens that include T3 should be considered. Oral T3 absorption is almost 100%, even when profound hypothyroidism is present. For patients who are able to take medication by mouth, a reasonable but unproven regimen is oral T3, 5–20 µg every 8 hours, plus oral T4, 25–100 µg/day. For patients unable to take medications either by mouth or nasogastric tube, comparable doses may be given intravenously. When clinical improvement is noted and the emergency has passed, T3 may be tapered and discontinued. Many other regimens have been suggested, including intravenous T4, 500 µg/day for 1–2 days, followed by 100 µg/day.

When refractory hypotension is present, stress doses of glucocorticoids should be given. Death from cardiac arrhythmias may occur 24 hours or more after an initial improvement in the myxedema crisis, and close cardiac monitoring should be continued for at least 48 hours.

Management of subclinical hypothyroidism

Most patients with a serum TSH level of 10 mU/L or above should be treated, as should pregnant women and those contemplating pregnancy who have serum TSH levels above the upper limits of normal for the assay used (generally 4.5–5 mU/L). Unless there are medical contraindications, a therapeutic trial with T4 is reasonable for symptomatic patients who have serum TSH levels of 5–10 mU/L. If no symptomatic improvement occurs, T4 may be safely withdrawn. Treatment is indicated for patients with minimal TSH elevation when a goiter is present and for individuals previously treated with radio-iodine for Graves' disease. Treatment guidelines are summarized in Table 5.3.

Several studies have shown a significant lowering of LDL cholesterol when patients with TSH levels of 10 mU/L or above are treated with T4.

TABLE 5.3

Guidance for treating and observing patients with subclinical hypothyroidism

Patient characteristic	Treat*	Observe*
Age	Younger	Older
TSH level (mU/L)	> 10	5–10[†]
Anti-thyroid antibodies	Yes	No
Symptoms	Yes	No
Heart disease	No	Yes
Goiter	Yes	No
Previous radio-iodine for Graves' disease	Yes	No
Pregnant or contemplating pregnancy	Yes	No

*There is still uncertainty regarding the correct course of action. In all circumstances, clinical judgment should take precedence.
[†]In symptomatic patients, consider clinical trial of T4.

Whether treatment of subclinical hypothyroidism improves wellbeing is uncertain, particularly for patients with a serum TSH level of 5–10 mU/L. Two small studies have shown improved symptom scores in more treated patients than untreated patients, but these studies included patients with much higher serum TSH levels.

Treatment of secondary hypothyroidism

Recognition of secondary hypothyroidism is particularly important because thyroid hormone accelerates the metabolism (inactivation) of cortisol. When thyroid hormone is given to an untreated patient with panhypopituitarism, cortisol levels fall, adrenocorticotropic hormone (ACTH) cannot rise and adrenal crisis may result. Glucocorticoid replacement therapy must therefore precede thyroid hormone replacement in patients with hypothalamic or pituitary disorders.

Monitoring difficulties. Monitoring thyroid function is more difficult in central hypothyroidism than in primary hypothyroidism. Serum TSH cannot be used to determine the adequacy of replacement therapy in these patients. Serum TSH commonly falls to undetectable values when T4 therapy is initiated, although free T4 concentrations are at or below the lower limits of normal. A combination of clinical assessment with free T4 measurements, which should be maintained in the mid-to-upper normal range, is used to monitor therapy.

Surgery in patients with primary hypothyroidism

Moderate or severe hypothyroidism should be corrected before elective surgery. Although serious complications can potentially arise when profoundly hypothyroid patients require surgery, emergency surgery can usually be performed safely without the need to render patients euthyroid beforehand. Careful attention must be given to:

- the choice of anesthetics
- judicious use of narcotics
- limited free water administration
- use of glucocorticoids for unexplained hypotension
- postoperative care of constipation.

Profoundly hypothyroid patients often do not develop a fever, even when infection is present, so extra vigilance is necessary. In general, mortality, intensive care stay, time to extubation, need for ventilation, electrolyte imbalance and duration of hospitalization in moderately severe hypothyroid patients do not differ from those of non-hypothyroid patients.

Key points – hypothyroidism: diagnosis and management

- Diagnosis of primary hypothyroidism is based on an elevated thyroid-stimulating hormone (TSH) level, which appears well before serum T4, free T4 or T3 levels fall below the normal range.
- Diagnosis of Hashimoto's thyroiditis is based on clinical features and the presence of anti-thyroid antibodies, usually with a high normal or elevated serum TSH level.
- Medical management of primary hypothyroidism is best achieved with T4, and should be carefully monitored to avoid hyperthyroidism.
- Profound hypothyroidism should be corrected before elective surgery, but urgent surgery can be safely performed even in moderately or severely hypothyroid individuals.
- Subclinical hypothyroidism should generally be treated if TSH levels rise above 10 mU/L, but first the condition must be distinguished from other causes of a mildly elevated serum TSH – a therapeutic trial is reasonable in symptomatic patients with serum TSH between 5 and 10 mU/L.
- Diagnosis of secondary hypothyroidism is especially important so that glucocorticoid therapy precedes thyroid replacement therapy (as thyroid hormone accelerates cortisol inactivation) to avoid consequent adrenal crisis.

Key references

AACE Thyroid Task Force. American Association of Clinical Endocrinologists. Medical guidelines for clinical practice for the evaluation and treatment of hyperthyroidism and hypothyroidism. *Endocr Pract* 2002;8:457–69.

Cooper DS. Combined T4 and T3 therapy – back to the drawing board. Comment. *JAMA* 2003;290:3002–4.

Pollock MA, Sturrock A, Marshall K et al. Thyroxine treatment in patients with symptoms of hypothyroidism but thyroid function tests within the reference range: randomised double blind placebo controlled crossover trial. *BMJ* 2001;323:891–5.

Roti E, Minelli R, Gardini E, Braverman LE. The use and misuse of thyroid hormone. *Endocr Rev* 1993;14:401–23.

Saravanan P, Chau W-F, Roberts N et al. Psychological well-being in patients on 'adequate' doses of L-thyroxine: results of a large, controlled community-based questionnaire study. *Clin Endocrinol (Oxf)* 2002;57:577–85.

Surks MI, Ortiz E, Daniels GH et al. Subclinical thyroid disease: scientific review and guidelines for diagnosis and management. *JAMA* 2004;291: 228–38.

Toft AD. Thyroxine therapy. *N Engl J Med* 1994;331:174–80.

Vanderpump MP, Ahlquist JA, Franklyn JA, Clayton RN. Consensus statement for good practice and audit measures in the management of hypothyroidism and hyperthyroidism. *BMJ* 1996;313: 539–44.

Normal fetal brain development requires thyroid hormone. Severe maternal hypothyroidism during the first two trimesters may result in irreversible neurological deficits, whereas the fetal thyroid may compensate for maternal hypothyroidism later in pregnancy. If treated soon after birth, inadequate fetal production of thyroid hormone does not usually cause neurological deficits, probably because of the protective effects of maternal thyroid hormone.

The state of heightened immune tolerance that exists during pregnancy prevents immunologic rejection of the fetus. Autoimmune thyroid disorders typically improve during pregnancy, only to worsen after childbirth. Postpartum thyroid dysfunction is surprisingly common. Thyroid dysfunction and thyroid nodules discovered during pregnancy require special attention.

Thyroid-related physiology in pregnancy

Maternal events. During normal pregnancy, the high-estrogen environment causes the concentration of thyroxine-binding globulin (TBG) to rise. As a result, serum total T4 and T3 concentrations (which primarily reflect bound T4 and T3) rise in early pregnancy, peak in mid-pregnancy and remain elevated throughout the remainder of pregnancy (Table 6.1). In addition, the placental hormone human chorionic gonadotropin (HCG), which is a weak thyroid stimulator, causes serum free T4 concentration to rise and the level of serum thyroid-stimulating hormone (TSH) to fall during the first trimester; both return towards baseline during the second and third trimesters.

Levels of serum TSH below 0.1 mU/mL occur in only 1% of uncomplicated pregnancies in the USA, but the prevalence is higher in other populations, such as individuals of East Asian descent.

Fetal events. The fetal hypothalamic–pituitary–thyroid axis matures progressively during pregnancy. At about 12 weeks' gestation, the fetal thyroid begins to trap iodine, and by 18–20 weeks it is working

TABLE 6.1

Thyroid-related physiology during normal pregnancy

Parameter	Level
TBG	Increased
T4	Increased
T3	Increased
TSH*	Normal to decreased
Free T4	Normal to slightly increased*
Renal iodide clearance	Increased

*First trimester; TSH < 0.1 mU/L is uncommon unless hyperemesis gravidarum occurs.
TBG, thyroxine-binding globulin; TSH, thyroid-stimulating hormone.

almost at full capacity. Fetal T4 levels rise during pregnancy and are comparable to maternal levels near full term. Maternal T4, and to a lesser extent T3, are transferred to the fetal circulation; however, the transfer is incomplete, as, at least in part, placental deiodinase enzymes inactivate the T4 and T3. This deiodinase activity, as well as increased sulfation of T4, explains why fetal T3 levels remain low throughout gestation.

Importance of iodine. During pregnancy, iodine requirement increases because of high renal iodide clearance by the mother and the fetal thyroid requirement for iodine. The net result is a fall in maternal iodine concentration. Borderline iodine deficiency before pregnancy can result in overt iodine deficiency and hypothyroidism during pregnancy. In areas with insufficient dietary iodine, goiters, caused by TSH stimulation, develop during pregnancy. Iodine supplementation can prevent these goiters. In areas with sufficient iodine, an enlarging thyroid gland during pregnancy must be considered abnormal.

The World Health Organization recommends 150 µg/day of iodine for adults and 200 µg/day for pregnant women. Until recently, iodine deficiency had all but disappeared from the USA, but now 15% of women of childbearing age and 6% of pregnant women have moderate iodine deficiency, with urine iodine excretion of less than 50 µg/L.

Unfortunately, many prenatal vitamin preparations in the USA and UK do not contain supplemental iodine.

Gestational hyperthyroidism

Gestational hyperthyroidism (HCG-induced hyperthyroidism) occurs in several settings:

- normal pregnancy (as described above)
- hyperemesis gravidarum
- hydatidiform mole.

Hyperemesis gravidarum is characterized by pernicious vomiting during the first 16 weeks of pregnancy and a loss of more than 5% bodyweight; spontaneous resolution occurs by mid-gestation. HCG stimulates estrogen production, which may cause nausea and vomiting in an uncomplicated pregnancy. Hyperemesis occurs when HCG levels are much higher than normal (or HCG has increased biological potency). Fortunately, this occurs in only 0.1–0.2% of all pregnancies. When HCG concentration exceeds 100 000 U/L, varying degrees of hyperthyroidism may result; generally they do not require therapy and do not have adverse maternal or fetal consequences.

Anti-thyroid drug therapy does not reduce the severity or duration of vomiting in hyperemesis gravidarum. Similarly, subnormal TSH levels during uncomplicated pregnancies do not require therapy. However, gestational hyperthyroidism must be differentiated from severe hyperthyroidism due to Graves' disease, which may be accompanied by vomiting (thyrotoxic vomiting), and does require treatment.

Hydatidiform mole is a rare complication of pregnancy. Extremely high HCG concentrations may be secreted by the tumor, resulting in severe hyperthyroidism. Hyperthyroidism abates once the mole is removed, but anti-thyroid drug therapy may be required before removal.

Graves' disease

Severe hyperthyroidism during pregnancy is uncommon, partly because it results in decreased fertility and partly because autoimmune disease generally remits to some degree during pregnancy. When severe hyperthyroidism does occur, it is generally due to Graves' disease. Toxic nodular goiter is rare in women of childbearing age in areas of iodine sufficiency. Some of the signs and symptoms of hyperthyroidism are found in a normal pregnancy (Table 6.2). True hyperthyroidism should be considered when a pregnant woman develops weight loss without vomiting, or muscle weakness, tremor, increased frequency of bowel movements or a pulse greater than 90 beats/minute.

Fetal complications of untreated moderate or severe hyperthyroidism include:
- increased spontaneous abortion
- small-for-age infants
- premature labor.

Maternal complications in untreated or undertreated women include:
- congestive heart failure
- pre-eclampsia
- tachyarrhythmias
- delivery-associated thyrotoxic storm.

Thyroid function in pregnant women with active Graves' disease should be tested monthly, using measurements of T4 or free T4, T3 or free T3, and TSH. Total T4 and T3 levels normally increase during pregnancy, and free T4 measurements are required to assess the degree

TABLE 6.2

Signs and symptoms of hyperthyroidism during pregnancy

In normal pregnancy and hyperthyroidism*	In hyperthyroid pregnancy only
• Heat intolerance	• Weight loss without vomiting
• Increased appetite	• Muscle weakness
• Shortness of breath	• Increased frequency of bowel movements
• Warm skin	
• Full pulse	• Pulse greater than 90 beats/minute
• Increased pulse pressure	• Tremor

*These signs and symptoms mimic hyperthyroidism, but are normal in pregnancy.

of hyperthyroidism. Ideally, free T3 should also be measured, although the measurement is less standardized. TSH suppression alone during pregnancy does not warrant therapy; however, therapy should be initiated when TSH suppression is accompanied by clinical symptoms and high levels of free hormones.

Graves' disease before or during pregnancy. Mild or subclinical hyperthyroidism during pregnancy does not cause adverse outcomes, and therapy is not required. However, untreated severe maternal Graves' disease can result in severe fetal hyperthyroidism due to transplacental passage of maternal thyroid-stimulating antibodies, which affect the fetal thyroid. The characteristics of fetal hyperthyroidism include:
- fetal tachycardia (generally greater than 160 beats/minute)
- fetal goiter
- advancing bone age.

Untreated fetal hyperthyroidism may result in fetal congestive heart failure or brain damage due to craniosynostosis.

Treatment. Guidelines for the treatment of Graves' disease during pregnancy are summarized in Table 6.3. The anti-thyroid drugs prescribed for moderate or severe maternal hyperthyroidism freely cross the placenta and treat fetal hyperthyroidism. Therapy is facilitated by the declining titers of thyroid-stimulating antibodies during pregnancy.

Methimazole and carbimazole have been associated with some very rare birth defects called methimazole embryopathy, which include aplasia cutis (a scalp defect that may require plastic surgery for repair), choanal atresia (a condition in which the nasal passages are blocked by bone or tissue) and esophageal atresia or tracheo-esophageal fistula. With this in mind, propylthiouracil may be slightly preferable, and is the agent of choice in the USA; women who become pregnant while taking methimazole are commonly switched to propylthiouracil. Methimazole or carbimazole is used in countries where propylthiouracil is not available, or if the last causes a minor allergic reaction.

The initial dose of propylthiouracil is generally 100 mg orally, two or three times daily, depending on the severity of the hyperthyroidism. When the free T4 concentration declines into the upper normal range, the dose should be tapered and, if possible, eventually discontinued.

TABLE 6.3

Treatment of Graves' disease during pregnancy

- Propylthiouracil may be slightly preferable to methimazole or carbimazole for anti-thyroid drug treatment
- Use the lowest dose of anti-thyroid drug that brings free T4 to the upper normal range
- Taper the dose of anti-thyroid drug as free T4 falls
- Anti-thyroid drugs can often be discontinued in the third trimester
- Consider surgery when very high doses of anti-thyroid drugs are required without adequate control of hyperthyroidism (propylthiouracil dose above 300 mg/day, methimazole above 30 mg/day or carbimazole above 45 mg/day), or when poor compliance or drug allergy occurs
- Use low doses of iodine (5–35 mg/day) to control hyperthyroidism in special circumstances
- Measure thyroid-stimulating antibodies in women previously treated for Graves' disease with thyroidectomy or radioactive iodine

Serum TSH may take weeks or months to return to normal, and dose tapering should not be delayed while waiting for this to occur. Combining anti-thyroid drugs with T4 is not recommended.

β-blockers may be used for brief periods during pregnancy, but prolonged use can result in intrauterine growth retardation, hypoglycemia, bradycardia and possibly respiratory depression, particularly when the dose of propranolol exceeds 160 mg/day at the time of delivery.

Radio-iodine (^{131}I) is strictly contraindicated during pregnancy. Radio-iodine given during the second trimester can cause fetal thyroid destruction. Other congenital abnormalities associated with the use of radio-iodine during pregnancy are rare and do not generally exceed the expected prevalence.

Surgery for hyperthyroidism can be performed in the second trimester, but this approach is generally reserved for patients who are either resistant or allergic to anti-thyroid drugs, or poorly compliant.

Surgery should be considered only when hyperthyroidism is poorly controlled with doses of propylthiouracil exceeding 100 mg three times/day, methimazole exceeding 10 mg three times/day or carbimazole exceeding 15 mg three times/day, or when patients are allergic to these drugs. β-blockers are generally administered for preoperative preparation, although iopanoic acid (not currently available in the USA – see Box 3.1, page 58), from 1 g/day up to a maximum of 3 g/day, is an alternative for patients with severe allergies to thionamides.

Potassium iodide is effective for moderate hyperthyroidism in selected cases. Although very high doses of potassium iodide may cause asphyxiating goiter in the fetus, doses of about 35 mg/day control maternal and fetal hyperthyroidism effectively without adverse consequences.

Neonatal hyperthyroidism. High-titer, thyroid-stimulating antibodies seldom persist until full term, but their persistence may be inferred when anti-thyroid drugs cannot be tapered without recurrent hyperthyroidism. Anti-thyroid drugs disappear from the neonate within hours, whereas thyroid-stimulating antibodies persist for at least 1 month. Hence, neonatal Graves' disease may appear 1 day or more after delivery.

Typical signs of neonatal hyperthyroidism include irritability, weight loss, tachycardia, congestive heart failure, hepatosplenomegaly and lymphadenopathy. Aggressive therapy with anti-thyroid drugs is essential.

Nursing with hyperthyroidism. The concentration of propylthiouracil in breast milk is low and does not adversely affect the infant's thyroid function; after appropriate discussion, propylthiouracil can be prescribed for nursing mothers. Higher breast-milk concentrations of methimazole (a metabolite of carbimazole) preclude full therapeutic doses, but a dose of 5–15 mg/day of carbimazole (equivalent to 3.3–10 mg/day of methimazole) appears to be safe in terms of neonatal thyroid and brain function.

Previously treated Graves' disease. Women in remission from Graves' hyperthyroidism may have mild worsening of thyroid function in the first trimester, but often do not need therapy. Postpartum hyperthyroidism (Graves' disease or postpartum thyroiditis; see below) develops in 33–70% of these women. Women previously treated for Graves' disease with radio-iodine or surgery may continue to harbor thyroid-stimulating antibodies, and measurement of these antibodies in this population is recommended. When the antibody titer is more than four times the normal level, the fetus is at high risk for hyperthyroidism.

Signs of fetal hyperthyroidism include a fetal heart rate exceeding 160 beats/minute and ultrasonographic evidence of fetal thyroid enlargement or inappropriately advancing fetal bone age. Fetal hyperthyroidism is treated by administering anti-thyroid drugs to the mother, who serves as a conduit to the fetus. Improved fetal thyroid function can be inferred from changes in fetal heart rate and fetal goiter.

Hypothyroidism in pregnancy

Severe hypothyroidism makes conception difficult. About 2.5% of pregnant women in iodine-sufficient areas have an elevated serum TSH level, but severe hypothyroidism is rare. Some clinical case series report congenital abnormalities in 10–20% of the offspring of severely hypothyroid mothers, perinatal mortality in up to 20% and neurological dysfunction in up to 50%. However, other studies report much more favorable outcomes.

The consequences of untreated subclinical hypothyroidism (normal free T4, elevated TSH) are uncertain, but it has been suggested that the IQ of the offspring may be affected. Euthyroid women with anti-thyroid antibodies are approximately twice as likely to miscarry as antibody-negative women.

Thyroid function testing is recommended in pregnant women with one or more of the following characteristics:
- a family history of thyroid disease
- a personal history of recurrent miscarriages
- symptoms suggestive of hypothyroidism
- a palpably abnormal thyroid gland
- known autoimmune disorders, such as premature gray hair or vitiligo.

Treatment. It is generally agreed that T4 therapy is indicated in women diagnosed with subclinical or overt hypothyroidism before or during pregnancy, although controlled trials are lacking. The goal of such therapy is to normalize the serum TSH level to within the lower part of the normal range.

When T4-treated women become pregnant, they often require an increased dosage. The magnitude of the increase is often greater than would be expected from the rise in serum TSH. For example, in a non-pregnant woman, an increase in serum TSH level from 2 mU/L to 10 mU/L might be normalized by a 25 μg/day increment of T4, but during pregnancy a dose increase of 50 μg/day or more is required.

Women with no remaining thyroid function require the greatest increase in T4 dose and may need up to an additional 150 μg/day (Figure 6.1).

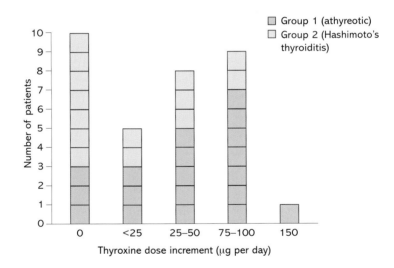

Figure 6.1 Increments in T4 dose required for a euthyroid state in women whose optimal doses were known both before and during pregnancy. Each square represents one woman. T4 dose increments less than 25 μg/day were achieved by having the patient take one extra 100 μg or 150 μg tablet each week. Group 1 is women with thyroid cancer (athyreotic), group 2 is women with Hashimoto's thyroiditis. Adapted with permission from Kaplan MM. *Thyroid* 1992;2:147–52.

Vitamins containing iron and other supplements used prenatally may bind to T4 and prevent its absorption, so it is important to administer the two medications at separate times.

It has not yet been established whether T4 therapy lowers the miscarriage rate in women with anti-thyroid antibodies.

Postpartum thyroid dysfunction

Postpartum thyroid dysfunction is the most common thyroid condition associated with pregnancy and affects 5–9% of women in iodine-sufficient regions. Postpartum thyroiditis may also develop after a spontaneous or induced loss of pregnancy, and the condition should be considered in the differential diagnosis of any disturbance of thyroid function identified in women within 1 year of giving birth.

Postpartum thyroiditis is an inflammatory autoimmune disorder considered to be a variant of Hashimoto's thyroiditis. The thyroid gland is diffusely infiltrated with lymphocytes; thyroid autoantibodies, particularly those against thyroid peroxidase, are present in almost all patients. Antibody titers generally decline as pregnancy progresses and then rise after childbirth, when the titers often exceed the values before pregnancy. Women who are positive for anti-thyroid peroxidase antibodies before pregnancy have a 35–50% risk of developing postpartum thyroiditis.

About 25% of women with type 1 diabetes develop postpartum thyroiditis, which also accounts for at least one-third of cases of hyperthyroidism in women with prior Graves' disease. Postpartum thyroiditis recurs in 50–75% of subsequent pregnancies after the initial episode.

Clinical course. Thyroid function in postpartum thyroiditis passes through several phases (Figure 6.2). In phase 1, transient hyperthyroidism typically develops 3–4 months after childbirth and is caused by the leakage of preformed thyroid hormone from the thyroid gland (destructive thyroiditis). The serum TSH concentration falls and 24-hour radio-iodine uptake is very low, as there is no TSH to stimulate its uptake. In contrast, radio-iodine uptake is normal or elevated in postpartum Graves' disease. Hyperthyroidism usually lasts for 3 months or less.

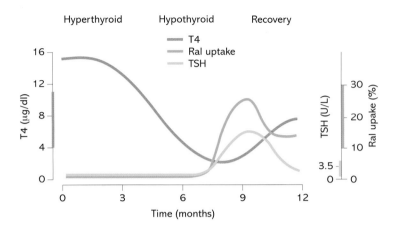

Figure 6.2 Typical time course of postpartum thyroiditis. The colored bars on each of the axes represent the normal ranges for thyroxine (T4; 4–11 μg/dL), radio-iodine uptake (RaI; 10–30%) and thyroid-stimulating hormone (TSH; 0.5–5 U/L).

In phase 2, thyroid function returns to normal as stored thyroid hormone is depleted, although the inflammation persists. Some patients remain euthyroid, but most pass through a hypothyroid phase (phase 3). Hypothyroidism may also occur without previous hyperthyroidism. It generally occurs 4–6 months after childbirth, but it can also appear up to 1 year afterwards. Return to the euthyroid state may take a year or longer (phase 4). Persistent or permanent hypothyroidism occurs in 25–30% of hypothyroid women with postpartum thyroiditis.

About one-third of patients with postpartum thyroiditis develop the classic pattern of hyperthyroidism followed by hypothyroidism. The other two-thirds are evenly divided between those who develop only hyperthyroidism or only hypothyroidism. Women with positive anti-thyroid antibodies may be more prone to postpartum depression, even if they are euthyroid and thyroid hormone is being administered.

Diagnosis. Postpartum hyperthyroidism due to Graves' disease (normal or elevated 24-hour radio-iodine uptake) must be distinguished from that due to postpartum thyroiditis (nil uptake). The correct diagnosis may be more difficult to make in a nursing mother. When hyperthyroidism is mild or minimally symptomatic, blood tests may be repeated after 4–6 weeks. Postpartum thyroiditis is the most likely diagnosis if thyroid function normalizes over this time.

Additional blood tests can prove helpful when hyperthyroidism is moderate or severe. The presence of thyroid-stimulating antibodies suggests Graves' disease, as does a serum ratio of T3 (ng/dL) to T4 (µg/dL) greater than 20.

Women with severe hyperthyroidism for whom these tests prove unhelpful should be encouraged to express and store breast milk so that they can undergo radionuclide scanning. Scanning with ^{99}Tc is preferable, because its half-life is shorter than that of ^{123}I. Nursing can recommence when the breast milk is no longer radioactive.

Treatment

Hyperthyroidism. β-blockers may be prescribed for symptomatic relief of hyperthyroidism in the first phase, but anti-thyroid drugs are not effective. Iopanoic acid may dramatically improve clinical hyperthyroidism by inhibiting conversion of T4 to T3, and may be used when clinical symptoms are severe. Glucocorticoid therapy shortens the time course of hyperthyroidism, but is seldom necessary.

Hypothyroidism. Experts disagree on whether, and for how long, to treat hypothyroidism due to postpartum thyroiditis. Profound symptomatic hypothyroidism should always be treated. As it is impossible to predict which women with mild postpartum hypothyroidism will progress to severe hypothyroidism, however, T4 therapy is generally recommended for all of them. Given the high risk of persistent hypothyroidism, this treatment should be continued until 2 years after the last child is born. When goiter and high-titer anti-thyroid antibodies persist, indefinite T4 therapy may be the wisest course.

Other approaches include administering T4 therapy only when marked symptoms are present, and limiting therapy to a specified period of time varying from 6 months to 2 years after childbirth.

Postpartum central (secondary) hypothyroidism

Central (secondary) hypothyroidism (see Chapter 4) may occur as part of the spectrum of postpartum hypopituitarism due to pituitary infarction (Sheehan's syndrome). Women who develop hypotension as a result of hemorrhagic complications at the time of parturition are at particular risk for this disorder. Hallmarks of Sheehan's syndrome are:

- an inability to lactate, secondary to prolactin deficiency
- failure of menses to return after childbirth, secondary to gonadotropin deficiency.

Another cause of postpartum central hypothyroidism is lymphocytic hypophysitis, an autoimmune inflammation of the pituitary gland that appears as a diffuse pituitary enlargement on MRI. Symptoms include those of hypopituitarism and those related to pituitary enlargement, such as headaches and visual field defects. TSH deficiency may be an early sign of lymphocytic hypophysitis.

Therapeutic approaches to secondary hypothyroidism are discussed in Chapter 5.

Thyroid neoplasms

Thyroid nodules may grow during pregnancy, and new nodules may appear at an accelerated rate. Thyroid nodules discovered during pregnancy are more likely to be malignant than nodules discovered at other times, so, although a reporting bias cannot be excluded, a fine-needle aspirate should be obtained from any newly discovered palpable nodules during pregnancy

Malignant or suspicious nodules can be safely removed during the second trimester. An alternative approach for smaller tumors that yield abnormal biopsy findings is prescription of thyroid hormone in suppressive doses during pregnancy and removal of the tumor after delivery.

There is no compelling evidence that pregnancy either stimulates or accelerates the growth of thyroid cancer metastases.

Women with thyroid cancer who require T4 therapy can be safely managed during pregnancy by maintaining serum TSH below 0.1 mU/L.

Key points – pregnancy and the thyroid

- Postpartum thyroiditis, an inflammatory autoimmune disorder, is the most common thyroid condition associated with pregnancy.
- Gestational hyperthyroidism (hyperthyroidism induced by human chorionic gonadotropin) may occur in normal pregnancy (subnormal thyroid-stimulating hormone), hyperemesis gravidarum and hydatidiform mole.
- Gestational hyperthyroidism associated with hyperemesis generally does not require therapy and does not have adverse consequences for the mother or fetus.
- Severe hyperthyroidism during pregnancy is uncommon, and is generally due to Graves' disease.
- Graves' disease during pregnancy is usually treated with thionamides; radio-iodine is strictly contraindicated.
- Untreated severe hypothyroidism during pregnancy may cause congenital abnormalities, perinatal mortality and neurological dysfunction in a high proportion of neonates.
- T4 therapy is essential in women diagnosed with hypothyroidism or subclinical hypothyroidism before or during pregnancy.
- In postpartum thyroiditis, transient hyperthyroidism is due to leakage of preformed thyroid hormone, and is followed by a longer hypothyroid phase, which persists in up to 30% of women.
- Anti-thyroid drugs are ineffective in the hyperthyroid phase of postpartum thyroiditis; therapy of hypothyroidism in this condition is controversial, but is generally recommended.

Key references

Alexander EK, Marqusee E, Lawrence J et al. Timing and magnitude of increases in levothyroxine requirements during pregnancy in women with hypothyroidism. *N Engl J Med* 2004;351:241–9.

Burrow GN, Fisher DA, Larsen PR. Maternal and fetal thyroid function. *N Engl J Med* 1994;331:1072–8.

Glinoer D. The regulation of thyroid function in pregnancy: pathways of endocrine adaptation from physiology to pathology. *Endocr Rev* 1997;18:404–33.

Lazarus JH, Kokandi A. Thyroid disease in relation to pregnancy: a decade of change. *Clin Endocrinol (Oxf)* 2000;53:265–78.

Mandel SJ, Cooper DS. The use of anti-thyroid drugs in pregnancy and lactation. *J Clin Endocrinol Metab* 2001;86:2354–9.

Muller AF, Drexhage HA, Berghout A. Postpartum thyroiditis and autoimmune thyroiditis in women of childbearing age: recent insights and consequences for antenatal and postnatal care. *Endocr Rev* 2001;22:605–30.

Smallridge RC, Ladenson PW. Hypothyroidism in pregnancy: consequences to neonatal health. *J Clin Endocrinol Metab* 2001;86:2349–53.

Epidemiology

The findings of autopsy and ultrasonography surveys show that thyroid nodules occur in more than 50% of people over 65 years old. Although only 10% of thyroid nodules are detected during the lifetime of those who have them, undetected nodules seldom cause serious problems, as about 96% of all thyroid nodules are benign. It has become increasingly common for thyroid nodules to be found when neck imaging studies are performed for other purposes. Larger nodules must be evaluated as if they had been discovered by palpation. Incidental nodules discovered by positron emission tomography (PET) are malignant in 25–40% of cases.

Thyroid cancer is the most common endocrine malignancy, although it makes up only 1% of all cancers, excluding skin cancer. It covers the whole spectrum of carcinomas, from the most indolent to the most virulent. The annual incidence of thyroid cancer in the USA is approximately 50–60 cases per 1 million women and 20–30 cases per 1 million men. In the USA, there are an estimated 25 000 new cases of thyroid cancer and 1500 deaths related to thyroid cancer each year. In the UK, about 900 new cases and 250 deaths occur annually. Because of the long survival of most patients with thyroid cancer, the prevalence of the disease approaches 1 in 1000 individuals.

Papillary thyroid carcinoma is the most common thyroid malignancy and has the highest 10-year survival rate (98%). This is followed by follicular thyroid carcinoma (92%), medullary thyroid carcinoma (80%), and anaplastic thyroid carcinoma (which seldom has long-term survivors). Large population-based surveys have not included thyroid lymphoma in the results.

Clinical presentation of thyroid nodules

Clinical assessment can sometimes suggest which individuals with nodules are at greater risk of developing thyroid cancer (Table 7.1). The clinician should be aware that patients with previous therapeutic head

TABLE 7.1

Findings that increase clinical suspicion of malignant thyroid nodules

- History of previous head or neck irradiation, particularly in childhood (predisposes the individual to both benign and malignant nodules)
- Less than 20 years old
- Male sex
- Nodule discovered during pregnancy (may be ascertainment bias)
- Hard, irregular or fixed nodule
- Associated with compression symptoms, vocal cord paralysis or enlarged lymph nodes
- Sudden growth not caused by hemorrhage or fluid accumulation
- Family history of thyroid carcinoma (medullary and possibly papillary)
- Family history of intestinal polyposis (familial adenomatous polyposis or Gardner's syndrome)

and neck irradiation are also at increased risk for primary hyperparathyroidism (serum calcium levels should be measured) and breast cancer.

Suddenly enlarging and painful thyroid nodules are generally benign and are usually caused by hemorrhage into a benign thyroid adenoma, although aggressive thyroid malignancies are occasionally associated with sudden growth and pain too.

Anaplastic thyroid carcinoma should be suspected if a pre-existing thyroid nodule grows rapidly and the size change is not caused by fluid accumulation.

A rapidly growing nodule in a patient with a history of Hashimoto's thyroiditis suggests a lymphoma of the thyroid.

The presence of multiple nodules (multinodular thyroid) does not exclude the presence of a thyroid malignancy, and larger nodules in a multinodular thyroid require evaluation.

Investigation of thyroid nodules

When a thyroid nodule is discovered it is important to determine whether it is malignant, while avoiding unnecessary operations. Whenever a thyroid nodule is detected by palpation, the physician must:

- perform a careful history and physical examination
- measure serum thyroid-stimulating hormone (TSH)
- refer the patient to a physician with experience and expertise in fine-needle aspiration biopsies.

A serum TSH below the normal range suggests a hot nodule (an autonomously functioning adenoma, defined by its enhanced ability to accumulate radio-iodine), which should be evaluated with a radionuclide scan (preferably ^{123}I) (Figure 7.1).

A thyroid scan is unnecessary when the serum TSH concentration is within normal limits, because a hot nodule is unlikely in this situation. Only 5% of thyroid nodules are hot, and these few need not be biopsied as they are almost always benign.

Although thyroid ultrasonography cannot determine whether a nodule is benign or malignant, it can provide the following information:

- the size of the nodule
- the presence and location of other nodules
- whether the nodule is cystic or solid
- which smaller nodules are suspicious and will require fine-needle aspiration.

In most cases, fine-needle aspiration biopsy is an indispensable procedure for distinguishing between benign and malignant nodules.

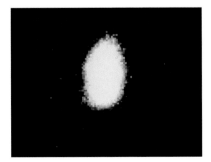

Figure 7.1 ^{123}I scan of hot nodule.

Current practice dictates that a fine-needle aspirate should be obtained from most palpable nodules. Exceptions may include:
- small soft nodules
- hot nodules
- smaller nodules that have been clinically stable for many years
- nodules less than 15 mm in diameter, particularly when multiple larger nodules are present.

Experienced clinicians may decide to biopsy a subcentimeter nodule if it is 'suspicious for malignancy' on the basis of its hard consistency. Thyroid nodules discovered at the time of radiological studies for non-thyroid imaging purposes should be biopsied if they are larger than 15 mm in diameter; smaller nodules should also be biopsied when high resolution ultrasonography is suspicious for malignancy. These criteria include a solid nodule with hypoechoic echo texture and one of the following:
- microcalcifications (Figure 7.2)
- an irregular border
- increased central blood flow to the nodule.

Non-palpable nodules must be biopsied under ultrasonographic guidance.

Fine-needle aspiration of the thyroid. Although most primary care physicians do not perform fine-needle aspiration, their patients often ask for information about the procedure and for help in interpreting the

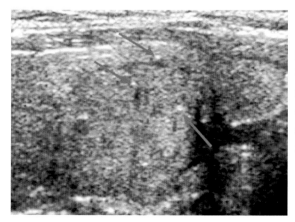

Figure 7.2
Ultrasonographic scan of a thyroid with a nodule showing microcalcifications (arrowed).

TABLE 7.2

Classification of results for fine-needle aspiration biopsy of thyroid nodules

	Percentage of biopsy results
Non-diagnostic	5–10
Benign	86*
Malignant	4*
Suspicious*	10*†

*Of diagnostic findings.
†Some laboratories include a separate category of 'suspicious for malignancy' (see page 115).

results. The procedure itself is relatively painless and brief, requiring only 10–15 minutes. Usually, but not always, a subcutaneous local anesthetic is administered. The aspiration is performed with a small needle, generally 25-gauge. Many clinicians repeat the aspiration with four or more separate passes to ensure adequate sampling.

Classification of fine-needle aspiration results is summarized in Table 7.2. A non-diagnostic biopsy occurs in 5–10% of aspirations and should be repeated, unless a fluid-filled nodule essentially disappears when fluid is removed.

Most of the nodules that are considered benign by fine-needle aspiration are characterized by monotonously similar thyroid follicular cells organized into large follicles that often contain abundant colloid. These benign-appearing biopsies are called macrofollicular lesions or colloid adenomas. Occasionally, an apparent nodule turns out to be Hashimoto's thyroiditis. The false-negative rate for a benign biopsy is about 1–2%, an acceptable percentage for a disease that is likely to progress slowly. However, all biopsied nodules should be carefully observed for continued growth. If a benign biopsy result does not provide sufficient reassurance for the patient, surgical removal of the nodule is advised.

A nodule classified as malignant by fine-needle aspiration biopsy will also be malignant on final pathological examination in 96–100% of patients (false-positive rate 0–4%). Papillary carcinoma, medullary carcinoma, anaplastic carcinoma, thyroid lymphoma and cancers that are metastatic to the thyroid can all be diagnosed by fine-needle aspiration.

Typical cytological features of papillary carcinoma include:

- overlapping cells with dense cytoplasm
- enlarged nuclei
- dense chromatin
- nuclear grooves
- nuclear pseudo-inclusions.

Follicular thyroid carcinoma cannot usually be diagnosed by fine-needle aspiration, because it does not have distinctive cytological characteristics. After surgical removal, when the final paraffin blocks are examined, follicular cancer is diagnosed if follicular cells invade through the capsule of the nodule or the blood vessels. If such invasion is absent, the nodule is a benign adenoma.

About 10% of thyroid nodules are made up predominantly of small thyroid follicles (microfollicles) and are considered suspicious. When removed surgically, 10–20% of these suspicious nodules prove to be malignant and are usually follicular carcinomas. The risk of malignancy in suspicious nodules rises to 40%, however, for nodules larger than 40 mm in diameter in men. The cytologist often describes these as follicular neoplasms or microfollicular lesions – intentionally ambiguous terms – until a surgical pathological diagnosis can be made. Unfortunately, examination of frozen sections at the time of surgery cannot make this distinction. Some suspicious nodules with follicular architecture turn out to be papillary carcinomas (follicular variant), and are diagnosed by their nuclear features on histological examination. Unilateral lobectomy is generally recommended for patients with nodules that are suspicious after fine-needle aspiration, when no other nodules are present.

Some nodules categorized as follicular neoplasms or microfollicular lesions by fine-needle aspiration prove to be hot nodules. Hot nodules are so likely to be benign that some clinicians override the fine-needle aspiration diagnosis of follicular neoplasm when a radio-iodine scan demonstrates a hot nodule. A radio-iodine scan is recommended when the serum TSH is low normal or low and the biopsy is suspicious.

However, some clinicians send all patients with suspicious biopsies for surgery.

Some cytologists utilize an additional fine-needle aspiration category called 'suspicious for malignancy'. Nodules that are suspicious for malignancy are more likely to be malignant than those which are just classified as suspicious.

Nodules that are predominantly cystic pose a dilemma. While they are not inherently suspicious, it is often difficult to obtain an adequate specimen by fine-needle aspiration. Nodules that decompress after fine-needle aspiration, and those in which the solid component is less than 10 mm in diameter, may be safely followed without surgery. When the solid component is larger than 10 mm in diameter, a non-diagnostic fine-needle aspirate is generally followed by an ultrasound-guided fine-needle aspirate. This latter technique facilitates needle entry into the solid portion of the nodule. Cystic nodules greater than 40 mm in diameter often re-expand after fine-needle aspiration. Surgery is often recommended for these larger cystic nodules, because of both cosmetic concern and the fear of missing a malignancy.

The indications for surgery are summarized in Table 7.3. Surgical removal of the lobe containing the nodule is the minimal operation recommended. Surgical indications for multinodular thyroids are considered below.

TABLE 7.3

Indications for surgery on thyroid nodules

- Malignant or suspicious FNA
- Larger nodule with repeated non-diagnostic FNA
- Continued growth of nodule after fluid removal and thyroid hormone therapy
- Symptomatic nodules (pain or pressure)
- Continued patient anxiety
- Some clinicians recommend that all nodules > 40 mm in diameter be removed surgically

FNA, fine-needle aspiration.

Non-operative follow-up and management after fine-needle aspiration. It is uncertain whether all thyroid nodules require ultrasonography as part of continued surveillance, but it does facilitate accurate measurement of nodules and the discovery of new nodules and is commonly ordered. Larger non-palpable thyroid nodules found incidentally require periodic ultrasonographic examination. The approach to follow for incidentally discovered, tiny (1–5 mm) nodules is uncertain, but follow-up ultrasonography after 1 year is often recommended.

The role of T4 suppressive therapy remains controversial. Only a minority of thyroid nodules shrink with such therapy, though T4 suppressive therapy may prevent the subsequent growth of nodules. Unfortunately, doses of T4 that suppress serum TSH to below 0.1 mU/L are also associated with thinning of the bones (particularly in estrogen-deficient women) and a high risk of atrial fibrillation (in elderly men). Partial suppressive therapy that decreases serum TSH concentration only to the lower limits or slightly below normal may also be effective in preventing nodule growth, while avoiding its harmful side effects, but is prescribed for only a minority of patients. When malignancy has been excluded by fine-needle aspiration, most clinicians give T4 therapy to patients with nodular thyroids who have had previous head and neck external irradiation, but T4 may also be used for some younger patients with larger nodules and for patients with pressure symptoms from their nodule. A repeat fine-needle aspirate should be obtained whenever thyroid nodules begin to grow. If the repeat fine-needle aspirate is benign and the patient has not been taking T4, it is commonly prescribed at this time to inhibit nodule growth. If a nodule continues to grow while a patient is taking T4, or if pressure symptoms persist, surgery is necessary.

Multinodular goiter

The term multinodular thyroid is commonly used to describe a thyroid with more than one nodule; when enlarged, these are called multinodular goiters. Many clinically solitary nodules are not truly solitary; ultrasonographic examination commonly reveals other thyroid nodules. The recorded prevalence of multinodular goiters is much higher when diagnosis is based on ultrasonography rather than on palpation, and increases with age. Multinodular goiters are more common in women then men, with up to 36% of women aged 49–58 years having nodules, increasing to nearly 50% at 65 years.

Pathogenesis. Although multinodular goiter is the most common endocrine condition in the world, little is known about its pathogenesis. It appears that heterogeneous populations of thyroid cells are present at birth in affected individuals. Some of these thyroid cells have an inherent genetic growth advantage and eventually develop into nodules. Many of these nodules are clonal in origin, while others appear to be polyclonal. Increased serum TSH level in regions of iodine deficiency and elevated levels of insulin-like growth factor 1 in acromegaly are two conditions that seem to accelerate the growth of thyroid nodules.

Clinical presentation

Hyperthyroidism. Most individuals with multinodular goiters have normal TSH and thyroid function. Occasionally, proliferation of autonomously functioning thyroid cells in a multinodular thyroid results in increased thyroid hormone production with a falling serum TSH. Subclinical and ultimately overt hyperthyroidism – a condition known as toxic nodular goiter – may develop. Radionuclide scanning then reveals either one or more discrete hot areas (Figure 7.3a) or diffusely heterogeneous uptake (Figure 7.3b), in contrast to the homogeneous uptake seen in Graves' disease (see Figure 3.1, page 43).

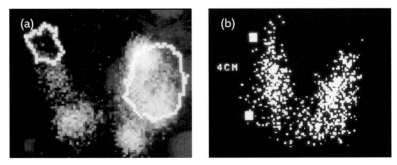

Figure 7.3 ^{123}I scan of toxic nodular goiter, showing (a) multiple hot nodules; (b) diffusely heterogeneous uptake.

Hyperthyroidism may develop slowly as autonomously functioning cells multiply, or suddenly if these cells are exposed to excess iodine (the Jod–Basedow phenomenon – see Chapter 2). Iodine-induced hyperthyroidism can be severe and protracted, as well as refractory to treatment. Iodine sources known to precipitate such hyperthyroidism include:

- intravenous iodinated contrast medium for computed tomography (CT), cardiac catheterization, angiography and intravenous pyelography
- oral iodinated contrast medium for abdominal CT scans
- amiodarone
- potassium iodide.

Potassium iodide has been distributed to individuals living near nuclear power plants in the USA in order to prevent thyroidal radio-iodine uptake in the event that radio-iodine isotopes are released during a catastrophic accident. If such an event should occur, it is likely that some cases of hyperthyroidism will develop after potassium iodide administration in people with multinodular thyroid glands.

When a patient with known multinodular goiter and low normal or slightly low serum TSH requires administration of an iodine-containing contrast agent, administration of anti-thyroid drugs (methimazole, 10 mg, or carbimazole, 15 mg, orally every 8 hours) before the contrast study may prevent subsequent hyperthyroidism. However, the effectiveness of this approach has not been tested systematically.

Local compressive symptoms and goiter. Compressive symptoms of large multinodular goiters may develop slowly over many years or more quickly when hemorrhage into a nodule causes sudden enlargement. Signs and symptoms of compression include:

- a sense of pressure in the neck (particularly when lying down)
- neck vein distention
- shortness of breath (sometimes misdiagnosed as asthma)
- difficulty swallowing solids (not liquids or saliva)
- hoarseness (due to vocal cord paralysis or laryngeal pressure).

Latent compression can be elicited by raising the arms over the head (Pemberton's maneuver), a useful maneuver for the physical diagnosis of compression due to goiter. Patients with latent compression develop facial plethora or erythema, dyspnea, distended neck veins or a sense of neck pressure. A low-lying nodular goiter may cause contralateral tracheal deviation. Progressive increase in neck circumference or collar size, without concomitant weight increase, is an important clue to a growing goiter.

Other problems of multinodular goiter include unacceptable cosmetic disfigurement and malignancy. The prevalence of malignancy in patients with multinodular goiter is about the same as in patients with a single nodule. Larger nodules and those with suspicious ultrasonographic findings should undergo fine-needle aspiration.

Treatment

Toxic multinodular goiter. The definitive treatment for toxic multinodular goiter is radio-iodine (^{131}I) following biopsy of suspicious nodules, or surgical excision. Although anti-thyroid drugs improve thyroid function, hyperthyroidism recurs when they are discontinued.

Bilateral thyroidectomy has the advantages of a more rapid return to a euthyroid state and removal of all the nodules. Traditional preoperative preparation for toxic nodular goiter consists of anti-thyroid drug therapy until the patient is euthyroid, but β-blockers alone can be used if a skilled thyroid surgeon performs the procedure. Surgery for multinodular goiter is recommended if biopsy findings are suspicious or malignant, or compressive symptoms are present. Surgery may also be an option when:

- there is radiological but not clinical evidence of compression
- the goiter is predominantly substernal
- the goiter continues to grow
- the goiter is cosmetically disfiguring to the patient.

Substernal goiters are best removed surgically, as biopsy is difficult and clinical observation without frequent CT or MRI scans is impossible.

Radio-iodine (^{131}I) is a simple and effective treatment for many patients with toxic nodular goiter. Hypothyroidism is less common after radio-iodine therapy for toxic nodular goiter than for Graves' disease, but it is still a common consequence of therapy. To speed the return to euthyroidism, anti-thyroid drugs can be given 1 week after radio-iodine and continued until the patient is euthyroid.

Euthyroid multinodular goiter. Once malignancy has been excluded, most euthyroid multinodular goiters require neither surgery nor medical therapy. Serial thyroid ultrasonographic examinations are useful to follow the size of individual nodules. Larger multinodular goiters require either CT imaging (without iodinated contrast) or MRI in order to exclude tracheal compression (Figure 7.4) and to assess thyroid size.

Radio-iodine therapy can decrease the size of large euthyroid multinodular goiters and relieve compression symptoms; worsening of compressive symptoms is rare. Most reports of effective radio-iodine therapy for symptomatic nodular goiter originate from countries with mild or moderate iodine deficiency, as decreased iodine intake usually increases radio-iodine uptake. A major potential drawback of such radio-iodine therapy is that many European countries require prolonged hospitalization for this therapy. In countries like the USA and the UK, where iodine intake is higher, it is uncertain whether radio-iodine therapy would be as successful. If radioactive iodine is used in these countries, a low iodine diet should be prescribed 2 or more weeks before therapy. Recombinant human TSH has been given to increase radio-iodine uptake and the efficacy of radio-iodine therapy as part of experimental protocols.

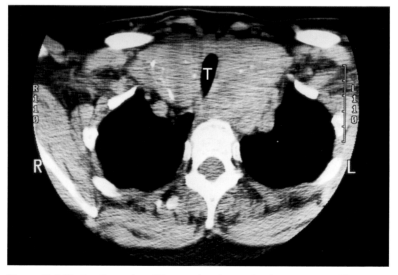

Figure 7.4 Obstructing goiter: CT scan showing tracheal compression (T).

Suppressive therapy (using T4) has limited efficacy in shrinking large goiters, but may help prevent the growth of smaller nodular goiters. The goal of therapy is a serum TSH at the lower limits of normal. If the serum TSH level falls below normal when modest (25–75 µg/day) doses of T4 are prescribed, thyroid autonomy should be suspected and the drug should be discontinued.

Hot nodules

An autonomously functioning adenoma, commonly referred to as a hot nodule, is defined by its enhanced ability to accumulate radio-iodine (see Figure 7.1).

Hot nodules make up only 5% of all thyroid nodules. Some hot nodules slowly progress to hyperthyroidism, whereas many others will not. Necrosis or hemorrhage into the nodule may self-limit progression to hyperthyroidism. Hot nodules less than 20 mm in diameter seldom cause hyperthyroidism, whereas those greater than 50 mm in diameter commonly produce hyperthyroidism. Excess iodide may precipitate hyperthyroidism in individuals with hot nodules, just as it may in individuals with autonomous multinodular goiters.

Pathogenesis. Hot nodules are clonal neoplasms that originate from a single parent cell. Several different biochemical defects can lead to cellular autonomy. Some hot nodules contain activating mutations in the TSH receptor, while others contain mutations in other proteins that lead to continuous production of cyclic adenosine monophosphate (cAMP) and cell activation.

Investigation. A hot nodule diagnosed by a suppressed serum TSH level and increased radio-iodine uptake is benign in over 99% of cases (a higher specificity for benignity than fine-needle aspiration biopsy). Although no longer ordered routinely to evaluate a thyroid nodule, a radionuclide thyroid scan should be performed when the serum TSH concentration is at or below the lower limits of normal to confirm that the nodule is hot. If a hot nodule is diagnosed, a fine-needle aspirate is unnecessary.

Therapy. A hot nodule with a normal or slightly suppressed serum TSH does not require therapy. A hyperthyroid hot nodule should be treated definitively with radio-iodine or surgery.

Radio-iodine (^{131}I) therapy of hot nodules has a low rate of long-term hypothyroidism and is simple, safe and effective, provided other worrisome nodules have been excluded by ultrasonography and fine-needle aspiration. Thyroid hormone production by the hot nodule suppresses serum TSH and radio-iodine uptake by the contralateral side (Figure 7.5); only the hot nodule concentrates the radio-iodine. Hypothyroidism occurs in only 4–5% of hot nodules treated with radio-iodine and with fully suppressed serum TSH, but is more common when serum TSH is low but detectable and contralateral radio-iodine uptake is evident on a radio-iodine scan.

Surgical thyroid lobectomy is also an effective and safe therapy for hot nodules. The risk of hypothyroidism after a hemithyroidectomy is low.

Direct ethanol injection is used in many European centers to ablate hot nodules. However, multiple injections may be required, and some patients experience considerable pain. Ethanol injection also may cause fibrosis and make subsequent surgery, if required, more difficult.

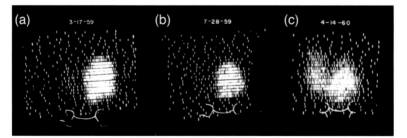

Figure 7.5 Radio-iodine therapy (^{131}I) of a hot nodule. The ^{131}I scans show suppression of the contralateral lobe and the appearance of contralateral uptake after radio-iodine therapy. (a) Pretherapy, the nodule concentrates iodine, but there is no uptake on the contralateral side. (b) Nodule has decreased in size. TSH is still suppressed, so there is no uptake on the contralateral side. (c) TSH is normal, and uptake can now be seen on the contralateral side.

Direct laser ablation is the newest non-surgical therapy for hyperthyroid hot nodules, and appears to be a promising innovation for future application.

Well-differentiated follicular-cell-derived thyroid carcinoma

Exposure to external radiation in infancy and childhood predisposes an individual to well-differentiated follicular-cell-derived thyroid carcinoma – either papillary or follicular thyroid carcinoma. This type of carcinoma has been a major problem in the regions surrounding Chernobyl in the former USSR (now Ukraine) in the years following the nuclear-power accident in 1986. Well-differentiated thyroid cancer is occasionally familial and may accompany genetic disorders predisposing to polyposis.

Papillary thyroid carcinoma is the most common thyroid cancer, constituting 80–85% of thyroid cancers in iodine-sufficient regions. Papillary thyroid microcarcinoma, defined as a tumor less than 10 mm in diameter, is found in 10–20% of autopsy specimens and is generally not of clinical consequence.

Pathogenesis. A mutation that generates the oncogene called *ret/PTC* is found in 10–40% of papillary thyroid carcinomas and may be an initiating event in malignant cell transformation. New data suggest that another gene, called *BRAF*, is mutated in 35–50% of papillary thyroid carcinomas.

Clinical presentation. Papillary thyroid carcinoma commonly presents as an asymptomatic neck mass, as either a thyroid nodule or an enlarged lymph node. It commonly metastasizes to lymph nodes, but these nodal metastases do not adversely affect the prognosis as they do in more virulent cancers, except perhaps in the elderly. Papillary carcinoma should be suspected when cervical lymph nodes display cystic degeneration. Papillary thyroid carcinoma is usually unilateral on physical examination, but microscopic contralateral disease is common.

Staging and prognosis. Many excellent staging systems for papillary thyroid carcinoma can be found in standard textbooks. In general, younger patients with smaller, non-invasive tumors have the best prognosis. A patient under 45 years old with an intrathyroidal papillary thyroid carcinoma, that is, a tumor that has not grown through the lining of the thyroid, can expect a 99% 25-year survival rate, even when lymph-node metastases are present. The prognosis is significantly worse if the following factors are present:

- extrathyroidal extension, defined as tumor growth into the surrounding tissue
- patient over 45 years old
- tumor greater than 40 mm in diameter
- distant metastatic disease.

Distant metastases may affect the lung, bones, brain and other tissues.

Fortunately, 85% of papillary thyroid carcinomas fall into favorable categories that have little effect on overall mortality. However, 10–30% of papillary thyroid carcinomas recur, including those with a favorable prognosis. The most common site of recurrence is the ipsilateral cervical lymph nodes. Although new diagnostic tools have made it possible to detect ever-smaller local recurrences, the clinical significance of some of these tiny tumor recurrences is uncertain.

Follicular thyroid carcinoma is the second most common thyroid cancer, constituting about 10% of thyroid cancers in iodine-sufficient regions, but a much higher percentage in areas of iodine deficiency, where large nodular goiters are endemic.

Clinical presentation. Follicular thyroid carcinoma generally presents as an asymptomatic thyroid nodule, but distant metastatic disease may also be its first harbinger. Bulky metastatic disease from follicular thyroid carcinoma occasionally causes hyperthyroidism, but it is not common. Bony metastases from papillary or follicular thyroid carcinomas are invariably lytic, seldom cause hypercalcemia and may be missed on radionuclide (^{99}Tc) bone scans. When suspected, conventional radiographs, or CT or MRI examinations, should be obtained. Pulmonary metastases from papillary or follicular thyroid carcinoma often remain asymptomatic for many years, despite tumor growth. Subsequent therapeutic decisions should take this feature into account.

Classification. Tumors previously classified as 'mixed papillary follicular carcinoma' behave as papillary carcinomas and are now classified as such. The follicular variant of papillary carcinoma also behaves like a typical papillary thyroid carcinoma and may have been misclassified in the past as follicular thyroid carcinoma. More precise diagnostic criteria mean that fewer follicular thyroid carcinomas are now diagnosed.

Prognosis. The behavior of follicular thyroid carcinoma ranges from indolent to extremely virulent. Tumor spread, when it occurs, usually does so through the bloodstream to the lungs and bones, and occasionally to the brain and liver; lymph-node metastases are uncommon. Follicular thyroid carcinoma with invasion of the tumor capsule but no vascular invasion has an excellent prognosis, with normal life expectancy in most, but not all, studies; pathologists may disagree about which carcinomas with capsular invasion alone are truly malignant. Follicular thyroid carcinoma diagnosed by invasion of only a few blood vessels has a variable but generally good prognosis, with a 10-year survival rate of up to 97%. When vascular invasion is extensive, however, 10-year survival is only 70%; many of these patients have metastatic disease at the time of diagnosis. Poorly differentiated follicular carcinoma (insular, solid or trabecular) has a poor prognosis, the 10-year survival rate being less than 50%.

Evaluation of well-differentiated thyroid carcinoma. Thyroglobulin is a protein produced by normal thyroid cells, benign thyroid nodules and well-differentiated thyroid carcinoma. When all normal thyroid tissue has been surgically removed and subsequently ablated by radio-iodine, residual thyroglobulin suggests the presence of metastatic thyroid carcinoma. Hence, thyroglobulin is an important tumor marker for well-differentiated thyroid carcinoma. Metastatic tumors that clearly immunostain for thyroglobulin are of thyroidal origin, a finding which may be helpful in localizing the site of origin of some adenocarcinomas. Serum thyroglobulin measurements cannot distinguish benign from malignant thyroid nodules.

Thyroglobulin release from benign and malignant thyroid cells is stimulated by TSH and decreases when TSH is suppressed. When searching for inappropriately elevated serum thyroglobulin, it is most informative to measure thyroglobulin when TSH is elevated. Serum thyroglobulin measurement in combination with radio-iodine scanning provides optimal information about residual cancer (Table 7.4), but it must be remembered that serum thyroglobulin elevations may persist for several months after thyroid surgery. Serum thyroglobulin cannot be measured reliably when anti-thyroglobulin antibodies are present, as occurs in up to 30% of patients with well-differentiated thyroid cancer. Therefore all commercial laboratories should routinely measure anti-thyroglobulin antibodies whenever they measure thyroglobulin. Disappearance of these antibodies over time is considered a good prognostic feature and suggests that residual cancer is absent.

Treatment of well-differentiated thyroid carcinoma. The appropriate care of thyroid cancer patients requires a multidisciplinary team with specific expertise in the diagnosis and management of thyroid carcinomas.

Surgery is the initial treatment of choice for patients with well-differentiated thyroid cancer. Bilateral total or near-total thyroidectomy, with appropriate nodal dissection, is the procedure of choice for all but the smallest papillary carcinomas. Surgical complications include unilateral or (very uncommonly) bilateral vocal cord paralysis, and transient or permanent hypoparathyroidism. The complication rate varies considerably, depending on the experience and technical skills of the surgeon. This procedure must be performed by surgeons with particular expertise in thyroid surgery.

Occasionally, the diagnosis of papillary thyroid carcinoma is not confirmed until the final pathological examination after a thyroid lobectomy. For tumors greater than 10 mm in diameter or with multifocal disease, a completion thyroidectomy should then be carried out because of the bilateral nature of this malignancy. After a lobectomy for follicular thyroid carcinoma in which the cytology was 'suspicious', treatment options range from T4 suppressive therapy for tumors diagnosed by capsular invasion alone to completion thyroidectomy or radio-iodine lobe ablation for more aggressive tumors. Follicular thyroid carcinoma is seldom bilateral.

TABLE 7.4

Evaluation of well-differentiated thyroid cancer with serum thyroglobulin and whole-body scanning

Serum thyroglobulin	Whole-body radio-iodine scan (low-dose radio-iodine)	Serum TSH	Conclusion/action
Detectable or elevated	Positive	Elevated	Residual thyroid tissue or metastatic disease; radio-iodine treatment
Nil (< 1 ng/mL)	Negative*	Elevated	No residual disease in > 99%
Detectable or elevated	Negative*	Elevated	Residual disease likely; check with ultrasound and, if negative, scan after therapeutic ^{131}I (shows site of disease in 10%)
Nil	Positive	Elevated	Consider interference in the thyroglobulin assay
Detectable or elevated		Suppressed	Residual tumor or residual thyroid tissue (probably malignant if discovered after radio-iodine ablation)
Nil[†] (< 1 ng/mL)		Suppressed	Disease free (80%, depending on disease stage)[‡] and residual disease (20%)**

*Exclude recent iodine contamination.
[†]After earlier radio-iodine ablation.
[‡]The number will vary depending on the population studied. A higher percentage will be disease free in a low-risk population; a lower percentage will be disease free in a high-risk population with previous metastatic disease.
**Serum thyroglobulin rises to > 2 ng/mL when TSH is elevated, which is indicative of residual disease.

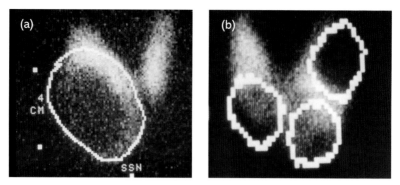

Figure 7.6 Cold thyroid nodule: (a) isolated; (b) multinodular thyroid with multiple cold nodules.

Radio-iodine therapy (*¹³¹I*) is the therapeutic mainstay for metastatic, well-differentiated thyroid carcinoma. The use of radio-iodine therapy in this situation might seem paradoxical, as most well-differentiated thyroid carcinomas are 'cold' on radio-iodine scanning (Figure 7.6). However, these tumors generally express TSH receptors, and can be stimulated to concentrate iodine when serum TSH is sufficiently elevated.

Small amounts of residual thyroid tissue are readily identified by radio-iodine scanning in most patients after so-called 'total thyroidectomy', and in this situation radio-iodine is often administered for three potential reasons:

- to facilitate subsequent follow-up with radio-iodine scans and thyroglobulin measurements
- to help prevent subsequent recurrences by destroying residual microcarcinoma in any remaining thyroid tissue
- to reveal unexpected distant metastatic disease.

There is general agreement that radio-iodine therapy should be given after total thyroidectomy for invasive disease, distant metastases or more advanced-stage disease. Papillary thyroid carcinoma is commonly treated with radio-iodine when it is larger than 10–15 mm diameter in the USA or 10 mm in the UK. However, the benefits of radio-iodine ablation for the smaller papillary carcinomas (which have a more favorable outcome) is controversial.

Radio-iodine scanning, ablation or therapy for patients with well-differentiated thyroid carcinoma requires an elevated serum TSH.

This can be achieved by either withdrawing T4 for 4–6 weeks or administering T3 instead of T4 for 4 weeks and then withdrawing the T3 for 2 weeks. A low-iodine diet should also be prescribed to maximize radio-iodine uptake. Iodinated contrast media must also be avoided for several months before radio-iodine therapy.

The whole body is scanned after administration of radio-iodine in order to discover cervical and distant metastatic disease, as well as residual thyroid tissue. The higher the dose of radioactive iodine used, the more likely unexpected disease will be seen (Figure 7.7). A scan should therefore always be performed after therapeutic or ablative doses of radio-iodine. Some clinicians prefer to scan the body after a relatively low dose of ^{131}I or ^{123}I, before ablative therapy. Patients with known or suspected metastatic disease should undergo a scan before therapy. Metastatic lesions visible on radio-iodine scans are amenable to therapy with radio-iodine, an advantage not shared by other scanning

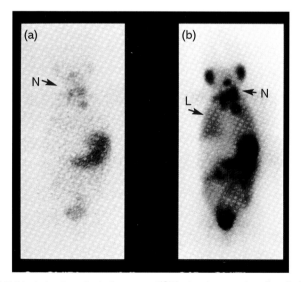

Figure 7.7 Whole-body radio-iodine scan (^{131}I) showing uptake of radio-iodine in the neck (N) and lungs (L), indicative of metastatic, well-differentiated thyroid carcinoma. (a) After low dose ^{131}I, scan shows uptake in the neck only. (b) After larger therapeutic dose of ^{131}I, scan shows extensive neck and pulmonary uptake. Originally produced in *Thyroid Today* 1993;16:1–9. Copyright 1993, Access Medical Group.

modalities. Unfortunately, not all well-differentiated thyroid cancers concentrate radio-iodine, and about 30% of those with metastatic disease will have negative scans even after the administration of high doses of radio-iodine.

Radio-iodine (^{131}I) therapy is generally considered to be safe and effective. Women must not be pregnant at the time of treatment and are advised to avoid pregnancy for 1 year after treatment.

The most common toxicity is sialadenitis, inflammation involving the parotid or submaxillary glands. This may lead to permanent dry mouth or recurrent episodes of painful salivary swelling. Permanent hypogonadism is rare, unless radio-iodine is concentrated in pelvic metastases close to the gonads. Tear duct blockage may also occur.

Higher doses of radio-iodine may require hospitalization for 1 day or more, depending on the state or country in which the treatment is given. Radiation precautions must be followed at home after high-dose radio-iodine therapy.

Thyroid cancer metastases, particularly those involving the brain and spinal cord, may grow when stimulated by TSH, with potentially life-threatening consequences. Such metastases must be identified before T4 withdrawal. They may be suspected when serum thyroglobulin is dramatically elevated at the time of TSH suppression; CT or MRI of the brain and spine should be performed in this situation.

T4 therapy is required for all patients after total thyroidectomy. T4 therapy is also prescribed to prevent tumor recurrence after surgery for well-differentiated thyroid cancer, as TSH is thought to stimulate tumor growth and recurrence, while TSH suppressive therapy is thought to inhibit growth and prevent tumor recurrence. For high-stage thyroid cancer, it is customary to use the lowest dose of T4 that can suppress the serum TSH level to less than 0.1 mU/L, and preferably below 0.01 mU/L. It is debatable whether full TSH suppression is necessary in all patients with less aggressive, lower stage, papillary and follicular thyroid carcinomas. In such patients, serum TSH is often fully suppressed for the first few years after diagnosis. For patients with no evident disease, a subnormal but not fully suppressed serum TSH level is a reasonable subsequent goal.

Follow-up. Many follow-up options are available after radio-iodine ablation. Serum thyroglobulin should be measured periodically in all patients after surgery for well-differentiated thyroid carcinoma. Detectable serum thyroglobulin after surgery and radio-iodine ablation suggests the presence of a residual tumor, which may be discovered after additional radio-iodine scanning, conventional scans or ultrasonography. Undetectable serum thyroglobulin (generally below 1 ng/mL) after injections of recombinant human TSH gives high assurance that no residual cancer is present.

In skilled hands, neck ultrasonography is the most reliable way of discovering nodal metastatic disease, which requires surgery in patients with papillary thyroid carcinoma. Pathological lymph nodes have a rounded appearance and a loss of central hilus or cystic change, and can be confirmed by fine-needle aspiration biopsy under ultrasonographic guidance or by measuring thyroglobulin on fine-needle aspirate washings.

Some clinicians recommend periodic whole-body radio-iodine scans as well. When the serum thyroglobulin level is elevated and the site of production is uncertain, the search for a residual tumor may include whole-body radio-iodine scanning after a large dose of radio-iodine, conventional CT or MRI of various anatomic locations, or whole-body PET or PET/CT scanning.

Surgical resection of symptomatic lesions should be performed whenever possible, even when distant metastases are present. Such surgery may require tracheal or esophageal resection and occasionally resection of metastatic foci in the central nervous system.

External-beam radiation is also effective for localized symptomatic lesions, particularly invasive neck lesions and inoperable bony metastases. Treatment of disseminated thyroid cancer that is either refractory or unresponsive to radio-iodine remains primitive. Current chemotherapeutic regimens have limited efficacy. Pulmonary metastases may remain asymptomatic for years, however, and when radio-iodine uptake cannot be demonstrated in these lesions, careful observation may be the most appropriate course of action.

Intravenous bisphosphonate therapy may be beneficial when multiple bony metastases are present.

Medullary thyroid carcinoma

Medullary thyroid carcinoma is a neuroendocrine malignancy of the thyroid parafollicular cells (C cells or calcitonin-producing cells). It accounts for about 4% of all thyroid cancers. Hyperplasia of the C cells is thought to be a precursor of medullary thyroid carcinoma. Medullary thyroid carcinoma cells are pleiomorphic and spindle shaped, and are often confused with a variety of other neoplasms, such as undifferentiated thyroid cancer. Medullary thyroid carcinoma may contain amyloid.

Etiology. Most medullary thyroid carcinomas are sporadic, but up to 25% are inherited in an autosomal-dominant fashion (Table 7.5). All patients with thyroid nodules should be questioned carefully about family members with thyroid cancer, hypertension or sudden death, because pheochromocytomas may accompany medullary thyroid carcinoma. Medullary thyroid carcinoma is generally bilateral in familial syndromes and unilateral in sporadic cases.

Genetic screening. Medullary thyroid carcinoma occurs in association with mutations in a proto-oncogene called *ret*. Analysis of peripheral blood for *ret* mutations is available through several commercial laboratories (www.genetests.org), and is advisable for all patients with medullary thyroid carcinoma after appropriate genetic

---

TABLE 7.5

Types of familial medullary thyroid carcinoma

- Multiple endocrine neoplasia (MEN) type 2a
  - Bilateral medullary thyroid carcinoma, pheochromocytomas, hyperparathyroidism (usually four-gland involvement)
- MEN type 2b
  - Bilateral medullary thyroid carcinoma, bilateral pheochromocytomas, marfanoid habitus, multiple mucosal ganglioneuromas of lips (bumpy lip syndrome), gastrointestinal tract and cornea; hyperparathyroidism uncommon
- Familial medullary thyroid carcinoma without other endocrinopathies

counseling. When *ret* testing is negative, the presence of bilateral carcinoma or associated C-cell hyperplasia mandates careful family surveillance by measuring serum calcitonin concentrations. When blood testing reveals a *ret* germline mutation, similar genetic testing should be done in all first-degree family relatives, provided they agree, after appropriate genetic counseling. If the same *ret* mutation is found and confirmed, total thyroidectomy is recommended.

Certain *ret* mutations predict aggressive tumor behavior. Multiple endocrine neoplasia 2b medullary thyroid carcinoma has a poor prognosis, and surgery should be performed as soon as the diagnosis is established. Children with less aggressive *ret* mutations may wait until they are 4–5 years old before undergoing surgery.

Diagnosis. The most common presentation of medullary thyroid carcinoma is an asymptomatic thyroid nodule or an enlarged lymph node. Almost all medullary carcinomas synthesize and secrete calcitonin, and some investigators (though not the authors) recommend routine serum calcitonin measurements in patients with thyroid nodules. In uncertain cases, positive immunostaining of the cells for calcitonin and an elevated serum calcitonin level confirm the diagnosis of medullary thyroid carcinoma. The diagnosis of 'poorly differentiated' or 'undifferentiated' thyroid carcinoma in a young patient should prompt a request for calcitonin immunostaining.

Prognosis. The prognosis in medullary thyroid carcinoma is variable. The 10-year mortality for patients with intrathyroidal medullary thyroid carcinoma is zero, but rises to 10% in patients with lymph-node metastases. With locally invasive and distant metastatic disease, the 10-year mortality reaches 35% and 60%, respectively. Many patients enjoy long asymptomatic periods despite having metastatic disease in the lungs and liver. Intractable secretory diarrhea and/or flushing due to carcinoma neuropeptide production sometimes accompanies advanced metastatic disease and may respond to octreotide therapy (a somatostatin analog). Secretion of adrenocorticotropic hormone from medullary thyroid carcinoma is a rare cause of Cushing's syndrome.

Treatment for medullary thyroid carcinoma is surgical, consisting of bilateral, near-total thyroidectomy, dissection of the central lymph-node compartment and exploration of the ipsilateral jugular lymph-node chain. Screening for pheochromocytoma is mandatory before surgery for medullary thyroid carcinoma, because hypertensive crisis may develop if surgery is performed on a patient with an unsuspected pheochromocytoma. External radiation therapy is employed for symptomatic metastatic disease and for residual non-resectable neck disease. Medullary thyroid carcinoma is not responsive to TSH, and T4 is given as replacement therapy rather than for TSH suppression.

Calcitonin is an extremely reliable tumor marker. Elevated serum calcitonin after surgery implies residual cancer, whereas a low calcitonin value is indicative of cure. Normal values for serum calcitonin are below 19 ng/L, but sensitive assays report even lower values in most normal subjects. After thyroidectomy, calcitonin should be nil. Carcinoembryonic antigen (CEA) is commonly cosecreted by these tumors and is an additional valuable tumor marker. The combination of falling calcitonin and rising CEA is a sign of tumor dedifferentiation and predicts a poor prognosis.

All residual cancer should be surgically removed whenever possible. When postoperative calcitonin is persistently elevated, it may be difficult to discover the site of production, even with progressive elevation. Common cryptic sites of calcitonin production include microscopic nodal disease in the neck or mediastinum, and microscopic pulmonary and/or hepatic metastases. Imaging studies to discover residual cancer include neck ultrasonography, and CT or MRI of the neck, chest and abdomen. More specific scans use labeled octreotide or radiolabeled anti-CEA antibodies. When serum calcitonin is relatively low and the residual tumor mass is small, these scans are often negative. Some clinicians recommend extensive surgical re-exploration of the neck in patients with medullary thyroid carcinoma when serum calcitonin is elevated and biopsies of the lungs and liver do not reveal metastatic disease.

Chemotherapy has limited efficacy and is generally not recommended for asymptomatic patients. Radiolabeled octreotide or anti-CEA antibodies have demonstrated limited efficacy, but neither therapy is commercially available in the USA or UK.

Thyroid lymphoma

Primary thyroid lymphomas are predominantly a disease of women, and occur most commonly between the ages of 50 and 80 years; they make up about 2% of all thyroid malignancies. About 2% of extra-nodal lymphomas originate in the thyroid.

Etiology. Most thyroid lymphomas develop from Hashimoto's thyroiditis over 20–30 years, and, although this transformation is rare, the risk is 40–80 times greater than in the general population. Many thyroid lymphomas are marginal-zone B-cell lymphomas of mucosa-associated lymphoid tissue (MALT). They grow slowly, have an indolent course and may show up in other MALT sites, such as the gastrointestinal and respiratory tracts, salivary glands and thymus. Diffuse large-cell lymphomas are derived from B cells and have a more aggressive course. Mixed tumors may occur. It is very uncommon for Hodgkin's disease, Burkitt's lymphoma or small lymphocytic lymphoma to occur in the thyroid.

Clinical presentation includes:
- hoarseness
- neck pain
- dyspnea
- dysphagia
- a choking sensation
- sudden enlargement of a neck mass
- growing bilateral lymphadenopathy.

A thyroid lymphoma is likely when sudden thyroid enlargement develops in a patient with known or presumed Hashimoto's thyroiditis and/or hypothyroidism.

Systemic symptoms, including fever, night sweats, loss of weight and disseminated disease with adenopathy, generally predict an aggressive large-cell lymphoma. In contrast, systemic symptoms are rare in MALT lymphomas.

Diagnosis. Thyroid lymphoma may be diagnosed by fine-needle aspiration, but a fresh specimen for flow cytometry is usually required.

Confusion may arise in well-differentiated lymphomas because of the presence of lymphocytes from coexistent Hashimoto's thyroiditis. When the diagnosis is uncertain, an open biopsy should be obtained.

Therapy for large-cell lymphomas generally consists of chemotherapy and external-beam radiation. Treatment of localized MALT lymphomas is more controversial. Some physicians recommend surgery alone, others recommend external-beam radiation or external-beam radiation after surgical excision. Disseminated MALT lymphoma generally requires chemotherapy. Surgical excision or tracheostomy is occasionally necessary for symptom palliation in more aggressive lymphomas.

Prognosis. Low-grade MALT lymphomas are rarely fatal, whereas tumors with a large-cell component, diffuse large B-cell lymphoma or advanced-stage tumors have the poorest outcomes.

Anaplastic (poorly differentiated) thyroid carcinoma

Anaplastic thyroid carcinoma is among the fastest growing and most virulent of all cancers. Most of these tumors develop in benign or low-grade malignant thyroid nodules, some of which may have been present for many years. A mutation in a specific tumor suppressor gene (*p53*, which normally facilitates apoptosis in damaged cells) is often found in these tumors, causing the damaged cells to divide and proliferate rather than be destroyed.

Anaplastic thyroid carcinoma commonly presents as a rapidly growing mass, often associated with symptoms of compression of neck structures and early development of distant metastatic deposits. When complete resection is feasible, surgical resection followed by external radiation and often chemotherapy may be beneficial. When resection is not feasible, as is most often the case, external radiation may control aggressive local neck disease.

Distant metastatic disease is unresponsive to current chemotherapeutic regimens, and death within 1 year of diagnosis is a common outcome. Paclitaxel may provide palliative benefit.

Key points – thyroid nodules and thyroid cancer

- Thyroid nodules are very common, but almost all of them are benign.
- Thyroid cancer is the most common endocrine malignancy, although it makes up only 1% of all cancers, excluding skin cancer.
- Fine-needle aspiration biopsy is indispensable for distinguishing benign from malignant nodules in most cases.
- The treatment for toxic nodular thyroids is radio-iodine (^{131}I) or surgical thyroidectomy.
- Papillary thyroid carcinoma (the most common thyroid cancer) often spreads to lymph nodes, but has an excellent prognosis in 85% of cases.
- Prognosis for follicular thyroid carcinoma is excellent when diagnosed by capsular invasion alone, and worse with increasing amounts of vascular invasion. The prognosis is variable for medullary thyroid carcinoma and very poor for anaplastic (poorly differentiated) thyroid cancer.
- Medullary thyroid carcinoma is familial in up to 25% of cases and may be part of the multiple endocrine neoplasia (MEN) 2 syndrome; close relatives of MEN 2 patients should be offered genetic screening.
- Surgery is the initial treatment of choice for patients with well-differentiated thyroid cancer and medullary thyroid carcinoma; radio-iodine ablation is often recommended for well-differentiated thyroid carcinoma.
- Thyroid lymphomas mainly occur in women and develop from Hashimoto's thyroiditis; high-grade lymphomas are treated with chemotherapy and external-beam radiation.

Key references

Ain KB. Anaplastic thyroid carcinoma: behavior, biology, and therapeutic approaches. *Thyroid* 1998;8:715–26.

British Thyroid Association. Royal College of Physicians. Guidelines for the management of thyroid cancer in adults. 2002. www.british-thyroid-association.org/guidelines.htm

Doria R, Jekel JF, Cooper DL. Thyroid lymphoma. The case for combined modality therapy. *Cancer* 1994;73:200–6.

Gharib H, Goellner JR. Fine-needle aspiration biopsy of the thyroid: an appraisal. *Ann Intern Med* 1993; 118:282–9.

Hay ID, McConahey WM, Goellner JR. Managing patients with papillary thyroid carcinoma: insights gained from the Mayo Clinic's experience of treating 2,512 consecutive patients during 1940 through 2000. *Trans Am Clin Climatol Assoc* 2002; 113:241–60.

Hegedus L. Clinical practice. The thyroid nodule. *N Engl J Med* 2004;351:1764–71.

Hegedus L, Bonnema SJ, Bennedbaek FN. Management of simple nodular goiter: current status and future perspectives. *Endocr Rev* 2003;24:102–32.

Heshmati HM, Gharib H, van Heerden JA, Sizemore GW. Advances and controversies in the diagnosis and management of medullary thyroid carcinoma. *Am J Med* 1997;103:60–9.

Mazzaferri EL. Management of a solitary thyroid nodule. *N Engl J Med* 1993;328:553–9.

Papini E, Petrucci L, Guglielmi R et al. Long-term changes in nodular goiter: a 5-year prospective randomized trial of levothyroxine suppressive therapy for benign cold thyroid nodules. *J Clin Endocrinol Metab* 1998;83:780–3.

Schlumberger MJ. Papillary and follicular thyroid carcinoma. *N Engl J Med* 1998;338:297–306.

Sherman SI. Thyroid carcinoma. *Lancet* 2003;361:501–11.

Singer PA, Cooper DS, Daniels GH et al. Treatment guidelines for patients with thyroid nodules and well-differentiated thyroid cancer. *Arch Intern Med* 1996;156:2165–72.

Useful addresses

British Thyroid Foundation
PO Box 97
Clifford, Wetherby
West Yorkshire LS23 6XD
Tel: +44 (0)1423 709707
Fax: +44 (0)1423 709448
www.btf-thyroid.org

CancerBACUP (UK)
3 Bath Place
Rivington Street
London EC2A 3JR
Helpline: 0808 800 1234
Tel: +44 (0)20 7696 9003
Fax: +44 (0)20 7696 9002
www.cancerbacup.org.uk

National Graves' Disease
Foundation (USA)
PO Box 8387
Fleming Island
FL 32006
Tel/fax: +1 904 278 9488
www.ngdf.org

Thyroid Cancer Survivors'
Association (USA)
PO Box 1545
New York, NY 10159-1545
Tel: +1 877 588 7904
Fax: +1 630 604 6078
thyca@thyca.org
www.thyca.org

Thyroid Eye Disease Charitable
Trust (UK)
TEDct, PO Box 2954
Calne SN11 8WR
Tel: 0845 121 0406
ted@tedct.co.uk
Especially valuable for
psychological support

Thyroid Federation International
797 Princess St, Suite 304
Kingston, ON K7L 1G1, Canada
Tel: +1 613 544 8364
tfi@on.aibn.com
www.thyroid-fed.org
Provides assistance with starting
thyroid patient organizations

Thyroid Foundation of America
One Longfellow Place, Suite 1518
Boston, MA 02114
Tel: +1 800 832 8321
Fax: +1 617 534 1515
info@allthyroid.org
www.allthyroid.org

Addresses of organizations in most
countries can be found at
www.thyroid.ca/English/
International.html

www.MyThyroid.com
A patient-oriented website

Index

acropachy 35, 40
adenoma (hot nodule) 43,
111, 114, 121–3
adrenal gland 16, 76, 81,
88
adrenocorticotropic
hormone (ACTH) 71, 90,
133
agranulocytosis 52–3
albumin 9, 12
alkaline phosphatase 36
amiodarone 21, 30, 44,
60, 62
anaplastic carcinoma 110,
136
androgens 20, 85
anemia 36, 79
anti-neutrophil cytoplasmic
antibodies (ANCA) 54
atrial fibrillation 31, 37
autoantibodies 21–2,
74–5, 103
to TSH receptor 22, 27,
41, 43, 100

β-blockers 48, 55, 61, 67,
99
binding proteins 9, 12,
20–1
biopsy 111–15, 135–6
'block–replace' drug
regimens 49–50, 56
bone mineral density 37,
83
breastfeeding 54, 100
bruits, thyroid 35

C cells 132–4
calcitonin 133, 134
cancer, thyroid 137
clinical presentation 110,
123, 124, 133, 135, 136
diagnosis 111–15, 133,
135–6
epidemiology 109, 123,
124, 135

cancer, thyroid continued
etiology 123, 132–3, 135,
136
in pregnancy 106
prognosis 123–4, 125,
133, 134, 136
residual disease 125–6,
129–30, 131, 134
treatment 126, 128–31,
134, 136
carbamazepam 20, 85
carbimazole 46–7, 48–56,
61, 98–9, 100
carcinoembryonic antigen
(CEA) 134
cardiovascular disease
hyperthyroidism 31, 37,
48, 61
hypothyroidism 72, 79,
89
central hyperthyroidism 30
central (secondary)
hypothyroidism 71, 72–4,
77, 82, 90–1, 106
chemotherapy 131, 134,
136
children
hyperthyroidism 36, 56,
67
thyroid cancer 57
cholesterol (LDL) 82, 89
cholestyramine 59, 62
clubbing 35, 40
complications see side
effects
compression
neck 118–19
optic nerve 34, 64, 65
computed tomography 24,
120
congenital abnormalities
98, 101
congenital hyperthyroidism
30, 100
contraindications 56, 99
contrast media 58, 118

cortisol 62, 90
creatine phosphokinase 79
cytokines 70

deiodinase enzymes 9–10
inhibitors 58–60, 61–2
diabetes 103
diagnosis
biochemical tests 12–22
hyperthyroidism 41–4
hypothyroidism 79–81
imaging 23–4
neoplasms 111–15, 133,
135–6
diet 10–11, 84–5
diplopia 34, 64, 65
dopamine 20

edema, periorbital 33, 64,
65
elderly people 26, 36, 64,
65, 84, 85
epidemiology
cancer 109, 123, 124, 135
hyperthyroidism 26–7
hypothyroidism 26, 70–1
nodules 27, 109, 117
esmolol 61
ethanol injections 122
etiology
carcinoma 123, 132–3,
135, 136
hyperthyroidism 27–30,
121
hypothyroidism 69–70, 71
nodules 117, 121
Europe 11, 48, 120
euthyroidism 14–17, 83,
120–1
exophthalmos see
proptosis
eye disease 27, 32–4,
38–40, 44, 63, 75

factitious hyperthyroidism
22, 44

familial dysalbuminemic
  hyperthyroxinemia 12
fetus
  hyperthyroidism 97, 98,
  100, 101
  hypothyroidism 101
  physiology 94–5
fine-needle biopsy 111–15,
  135–6
follicular carcinoma 109,
  114, 124–5, 126
free hormone levels
  (T3/T4) 9, 12, 18, 20–1,
  79, 82
free T4 index (FTI) 18

genetic factors
  neoplasms 121, 123,
  132–3, 136
  TSH receptor mutations
  30, 71
glucocorticoids 14, 48, 62,
  65, 89, 90, 105
goiter 10, 27, 31, 70
  multinodular 27, 42,
  46–7, 116–21
granulocyte colony-
  stimulating factor 53, 70
granulocytopenia 36, 52–3
Graves' disease
  clinical presentation
  31–6, 97–8
  complications 36–40, 97
  diagnosis 23, 41, 43, 105
  epidemiology 27
  etiology 27
  postpartum 101, 104–5
  in pregnancy 50, 96–101
  treatment 36, 44–62,
  66–7, 98–101

Hashimoto's
  encephalopathy 76
Hashimoto's thyroiditis 70,
  74–6, 81, 83–8, 102, 135
  see also thyroiditis,
  postpartum
hematologic abnormalities
  36, 52–3, 79
heparin 20–1
heterophilic antibodies 16

homocysteine 79
human chorionic
  gonadotropin (HCG) 29,
  94, 96
Hurthle cells 74
hydatidiform mole 96
hydrocortisone 62, 90
hyperemesis gravidarum 96
hyperparathyroidism 110
hyperthyroidism 38, 66
  clinical presentation 19,
  31–6, 97–8, 117–18
  complications 36–40, 97
  diagnosis 14–15, 23, 41–4
  epidemiology 26–7
  etiology 27–30, 121
  postpartum 101, 103,
  104–5
  in pregnancy 50, 96–101
  treatment 36, 44–67, 96,
  98–101, 105, 119
hypokalemia 38
hypotension 61, 89
hypothalamus 10, 71, 82
hypothyroidism 77, 92
  clinical presentation 18,
  19, 72–6
  complications 76–7, 91,
  101
  diagnosis 14–15, 21, 22,
  79–81
  epidemiology 26, 70–1
  etiology 69–70, 71
  iatrogenic 50, 55, 56–7,
  69, 119, 122
  postpartum 104, 105–6
  in pregnancy 85, 94,
  101–3
  treatment 83–91, 102–3,
  105

immunosuppression 63, 65
intensive care 20, 84, 89
iodine
  hyperthyroidism 29, 44,
  61, 118
  hypothyroidism 69, 70
  metabolism 9, 10–12, 22,
  95
  in pregnancy 95–6, 100
  therapy 60, 62, 67, 100

iodine continued
  see also radio-iodine
  therapy
iopanoic acid 58–60, 61–2,
  67, 100, 105

Jod–Basedow phenomenon
  118

laser ablation 123
lithium 61, 70
liver function tests 36, 53–4
lymph nodes 123, 131
lymphocytic thyroiditis
  chronic see Hashimoto's
  thyroiditis
  subacute 29, 43–4
lymphoma 135–6

magnetic resonance
  imaging 24, 44
MALT lymphoma 135, 136
medullary carcinoma 132–4
metastasis 123, 124, 125,
  129, 130, 133, 134, 136
methimazole 46–7, 48–56,
  61, 98–9, 100
microcalcifications 112
multiple endocrine
  neoplasia (MEN) 132
myxedema crisis 76, 88–9
myxedema, pretibial 34–5,
  40

neonatal hyperthyroidism
  30, 100
nodular disease 137
  clinical presentation
  109–10, 117–19
  diagnosis 23–4, 81,
  111–15, 121
  epidemiology 27, 109,
  117
  etiology 117, 121
  hot nodule 43, 111, 114,
  121–3
  multinodular 27, 42,
  46–7, 116–21
  in pregnancy 106
  treatment 46–7, 57–8,
  115–16, 119–21, 122–3

non-thyroidal illness 12, 19–20
NOSPECS mnemonic 34
nuclear accidents 118, 123

octreotide 133, 134
ophthalmopathy 27, 32–4, 38–40, 44, 63, 75
osteoporosis 37, 83

paclitaxel 136
papillary carcinoma 109, 114, 123–4, 125, 126, 128
paralysis 38
patients, information for 46–7, 52, 57
Pemberton's maneuver 118
perchlorate discharge test 22
perchlorate therapy 61
phenytoin 20, 85
pheochromocytoma 132, 134
pituitary gland
  feedback control 10
  hypopituitarism 13, 14–15, 71, 82, 90, 106
  tumors 30, 42
plasmapheresis 62
postpartum disease 29, 43–4, 94, 103–6
postviral thyroiditis 29, 43, 48
pregnancy 107
  hyperthyroidism 50, 96–101
  hypothyroidism 85, 94, 101–3
  neoplasms 106
  physiology 94–5
  postpartum disease 29, 43–4, 94, 103–6
prolactin 80
propranolol 61, 67
proptosis 39, 64, 65, 75
propylthiouracil (PTU) 46–7, 48–56, 61, 98–9, 100

radio-iodine therapy
  hyperthyroidism 45, 46, 47–8, 54–8, 63, 99
  neoplasms 119, 120, 122, 128–30
radionuclide scans
  hyperthyroidism 23, 41–4, 105
  neoplasms 23, 111, 117, 127, 128, 129–30, 131
radiotherapy (external-beam) 57, 69, 110, 131, 136
ret proto-oncogene 132–3

sex-hormone-binding globulin 36
Sheehan's syndrome 106
side effects
  perchlorate 61
  radio-iodine 47, 57–8, 130
  surgery 47, 66–7, 126
  thionamides 47, 51–4, 98
smoking 38
sodium 79
sodium ipodate 58–60, 61–2
steroids 20, 36, 85
  see also glucocorticoids
'stunning' 57
subclinical disease
  hyperthyroidism 26, 30–1, 41, 63–5
  hypothyroidism 70–1, 77, 81–2, 89–90
surgery
  eye disease 63
  hyperthyroidism 45, 46–7, 48, 66–7, 99–100
  in hypothyroid patients 91
  neoplasms 114, 115, 119, 122, 126, 131, 134, 136

T3 resin uptake test 18
T3 (triiodothyronine)
  hyperthyroidism 41
  hypothyroidism 79, 80, 81
  physiology 9–10, 94
  pregnancy 94
  tests for 12, 18, 20, 21
  therapy 84, 89

T4 (L-thyroxine)
  hyperthyroidism 14–15, 41
  hypothyroidism 14–15, 80, 81, 82
  physiology 9–10, 94
  pregnancy/postpartum 94, 102–3, 104, 105
  replacement therapy 49–50, 56, 83–8, 89–90, 102–3, 105
  suppressive therapy 116, 121, 130
  tests for 12, 14–17, 18, 20, 21
[99]technecium scans 23
thionamide drugs 45, 46–7, 48–56, 61, 67, 98–9, 100
thyroglobulin 9, 22, 44, 125–6, 131
  antibodies to 22
thyroid-binding globulin (TBG) 9, 94
thyroid-binding prealbumin 9
thyroidectomy
  see surgery
thyroid function tests 12–22, 24
  hyperthyroidism 14–15, 30–1, 41
  hypothyroidism 14–15, 79–80, 81, 82
  neoplasms 111, 127
  in pregnancy 94–5, 97–8
thyroid-hormone-binding ratio (THBR) 18
thyroiditis
  autoimmune 69–70, 74–6, 79–81, 83–8
  destructive 29–30, 42, 43–4, 48, 54
  lymphocytic 29, 43–4
  postpartum 29, 43, 103–5
thyroid peroxidase 9
  antibodies to 21, 103
thyroid-stimulating hormone see TSH

thyroid-stimulating
  hormone receptor
  antibodies to 22, 27, 41,
  43, 100
  mutations 30, 71
thyrotoxicosis see
  hyperthyroidism
thyrotoxic storm 37–8,
  61–2
thyrotropin-releasing
  hormone (TRH) 10, 21,
  82
L-thyroxine
  see T4
total hormone levels
  (T3/T4) 9, 12, 18
trachea 119, 120
triiodothyronine
  see T3

TSH (thyroid-stimulating
  hormone)
  hyperthyroidism 14–15,
  30–1, 41
  hypothyroidism 14–15,
  71, 79, 81, 82, 83, 87–8
  neoplasms 111, 127, 129,
  130
  physiology 9, 10, 94
  pituitary tumors 30, 42
  pregnancy 94, 104
  recombinant 120
  tests for 13–17, 18–20
UK
  epidemiology 7, 26, 109
  radionuclide scans 41
  treatment 48, 56, 58, 120
ultrasonography 23–4, 44,
  81, 111, 112, 116, 131

USA
  epidemiology 7, 26,
  109
  iodine deficiency 69,
  95
  treatment 47, 48, 56, 58,
  120

vitamin B$_{12}$ 75–6
vitamins, and T4 therapy
  84–5, 103
vomiting 36, 96
von Basedow's disease
  see Graves' disease

weight changes 32, 36,
  74
white blood cell count
  53

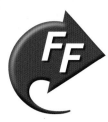